What students are saying:

"I was accepted to 5 out of 6! - F. Edward Herbert School of Medicine - University of Vermont College of Medicine - Cooper Medical School of Rowan University - Oakland University of William Beaumont School of Medicine - Rutgers Robert Wood Johnson Medical School." – Ada

"Just wanted to drop you a line and let you know that I was accepted into all three schools (Queen's, Mac and U of T) but will be accepting U of T. Thanks again for all the help in the process [application review, CASPer prep & interview prep] and I look forward to seeing you around campus / hospitals in the near future. Cheers, " – Mandolin

"I got accepted to UC Davis, Georgetown, UC Riverside (full scholarship - matriculating), Loma Linda, and UCLA. I've thus far recommended your site to anyone I meet." – Marysia

"Just wanted to drop you a line and let you know that I was accepted into all three schools (Queen's, Mac and U of T) but will be accepting U of T. Thanks again for all the help in the process [application review, CASPer prep & interview prep] and I look forward to seeing you around campus / hospitals in the near future. Cheers, " – Sameer

"Hello, The interviews went great, thanks again for all the help [with CASPer & interview prep]! I was accepted to McMaster, Queen's, and NOSM [medical schools]. Thanks again, " – Jesse

"Thank you for your assistance in preparing me with the CASPer and MMI interviews! I wanted to let you know that I was accepted at Robert Wood Johnson Medical School! Please extend my thanks to the instructors who helped me prepare. Thanks again," – Jason

"I was accepted to the University of Vermont (UVM) and Quinnipiac (Frank H. Netter MD School of Medicine at Quinnipiac University) and will be going to UVM in the fall, which I'm very excited about! I appreciate all the help BeMo provided me in preparing for my interview!!" – Danielle

"Thanks for checking in. Yes, the interviews went really well - I got into all the universities I interviewed at (Toronto, McMaster, and Northern)!" – Megan

"I have heard back from all the schools I applied to. I was accepted at 6 different veterinary schools: Texas A&M, Midwestern, Mississippi State, Oklahoma State, Penn, and Cornell. I was initially waitlisted at Penn and Cornell. Texas A&M conducted an MMI style interview, while Midwestern, Mississippi State, and Penn had traditional interviews. I will be attending my in-state school, Texas A&M, starting in August. Thank you for all your help!" – Callie

"Thanks for the message. The application process went really well, and I am excited to be attending Columbia University College of Physicians and Surgeons in the fall. Thank you for your help," – Andy

"Good News! I was accepted to all three medical schools where I interviewed: University of Toronto, University of Ottawa, and Albert Einstein College of Medicine. I have officially accepted my offer to U of T... Thanks again for all your help! I was very pleased with the service I received." – Joanna

"Hello! My interviews went great actually. I was accepted at NYMC and UMass Medical School, both of which had MMI interview format. I will be attending UMass in the fall. Both my mock interviews gave me really good preparation and the interviewers were wonderful! So I certainly owe a lot of credit to BeMo for helping me reach my goals :) I'd be happy to write a testimonial, etc. Thank you," – Nate

"I hope you are well. I've received acceptances from the University of Toronto, University of Saskatchewan, and University of British Columbia and I'm on the waitlisted at the University of Ottawa. I think BeMo definitely helped prepare me! I'm very grateful for those who helped me improve and prepare." – Saloni

"Thank you for your email. I'll be attending UCSD in the fall. Thank you for the support and resources!" – Jessica

BeMo's Ultimate Guide to Medical School Admissions in the U.S. and Canada

LEARN TO PLAN IN ADVANCE, MAKE YOUR
APPLICATIONS STAND OUT, ACE YOUR CASPER TEST,
& MASTER YOUR MULTIPLE MINI INTERVIEWS

BeMo Academic Consulting Inc.

ISBN: 1530790107
ISBN 13: 9781530790104

LIST OF CONTRIBUTING AUTHORS

Dr. Helena L. Frishtak, B.Sc., MD

Dr. Izu Ibe, H.B.Sc., MD

Dr. Perry Guo, M.D.

Dr. Natalie Lidster, H.B.Sc., MD

Dr. Janet McMordie, B.Sc., M.Sc., MD

Dr. Lauren Prufer, H.B.Sc. MD

Dr. Ashley White, H.B.Sc., MPH, MD

Dan Wang, B.Eng., M.S, MBA, MD(c)

Ms. Lindsay McCaw, H.B.Sc., M.Sc.
Editor

Ms. Ronza Nissan, H.B.A., MA

Dr. Mo Bayegan, H.B.Sc., DC

Dr. Behrouz Moemeni, H.B.Sc., Ph.D.

Contents

Foreword

First of all, CONGRATULATIONS for making the commitment to educate yourself to become not only a competitive medical school applicant, but also a better person, and as a result a better physician in the future. The fact that you have purchased this book tells us that you are the type of person who is willing to invest in yourself and learn more. The world rewards individuals who continuously seek to educate themselves because "knowledge is power." Before we get into the details, we need to set the record straight about why you should listen to us, what this book is all about, and who this book is for and who it is NOT for.

Here's A Bit About Us: BeMo Academic Consulting ("BeMo") BeMoAcademicConsulting.com

We're an energetic academic consulting firm, comprised of a team of researchers and professionals, who use a proven evidence-based and scientific approach to help prospective students with career path development and admissions to undergraduate, graduate and professional programs (e.g. medicine, law, dentistry, pharmacy, etc.)

We believe your education is your most valuable asset and learning how to become a great future professional or scholar doesn't need to be complicated. We also believe that every student deserves access to higher education, regardless of his or her social status or cultural background. However, in our opinion, most of the current admissions practices, tools and procedures are not necessarily fair and for the most part out-dated and more importantly, remain scientifically unproven.

Our goal is to create insanely useful (and scientifically sound) programs and tools that work and provide more than just some trivial information like the other "admissions consulting companies" out there! We want to make sure everyone has a fair chance of admissions to highly competitive professional programs despite the current admissions practices.

We do whatever it takes to come up with creative solutions...and then implement like mad scientists. We're passionate about mentoring our students and obsessed with delivering insanely useful educational programs and we go where others dare not to explore.

Why should you listen to us?

Our primary area of focus is the extremely competitive field of medical school admissions. We have an exceptional team of medical doctors, scholars and scientists who have served as former admissions committee members (visit our website, BeMoAcademicConsulting.com, to learn more about our admissions experts). To give you an idea, each year we help hundreds of students gain admission to top medical schools. What we are about to share is based on what we have learned in our much sought-after one-on-one coaching programs. What we offer works and it works consistently. Our programs are in high demand and we are certain they will also work for you!

Why did we write this book?

There's so much misinformation online and offline. From online pre-med forums to pre-med clubs and even some university guidance counselors. While some of these sources are well intended (not all are well-intended), the level of misinformation is astounding. For example, in our opinion, most online pre-med forums cannot be trusted because it is not clear who the authors are, what motivates them and importantly whether or not such sources are credible. To make matters worse, some of these forums offer 'sponsorship opportunities' to companies, which puts them in a financial conflict of interest. Most pre-med clubs are also to be avoided because often times they also form financial relationships with companies to support their operations and as such they provide one-sided information. Additionally, most books out there are incomplete and tend to have a narrow focus on teaching you 'tricks' about applications or multiple mini interviews. They do not focus on the big picture that is essential to your success, both as an applicant and as a future doctor.

What is this book about?

This book is about the big picture, which is how to develop into a mature, professional, ethical and knowledgeable individual, which is essential to becoming a future medical doctor. While we spend a considerable amount of time walking you through specific instructions about your application to medical school, it is important to always remain focused on the big picture. The book is designed to teach you everything you need to know about the medical school admission process, and how to make your application stand out. We will give you an overview of each chapter in the introductory section, but briefly, in this book we'll cover various topics ranging from the rationale behind the admission process, planning in advance, filling out applications, and we will even discuss strategies that will help you ace your CASPer test and interview.

Who is this book for and who is it NOT for?

If you're just starting to think about or plan for medical school (e.g. you are in early undergraduate studies, or late high school, or a nontraditional candidate who has just decided to pursue medicine), then this is perfect for you. If you have already successfully planned your path to medical school and/or are in the application process, then specific chapter on how to prepare your application, how to ace the CASPer test, and finally the chapter about acing medical school interviews, will be extremely useful. No matter where you are starting, this book has something for you, provided that you are willing to put in the hard work and invest in yourself. Getting into medical school is not easy. Nor is being a medical doctor. **In fact, getting into medical school is very difficult and**

very expensive in terms of time, money and energy. And importantly, we do NOT share any quick 'tricks' and 'shortcuts' or 'insider' scoops like some of the other books out there. **Therefore, this book is NOT for anyone who is looking for an easy, cheap, shortcut to get into medical school.**

We do not share any such trick or shortcuts because:

A) There are no tricks or insider info that can help you, because you cannot trick your way to becoming a mature, ethical professional. Rather, you must put in long hours of self-training. Think of it this way, just like a professional athlete trains for years (on average ten years, hence the "ten-year rule" to mastery) to get to that level of proficiency, wouldn't it make sense that our future doctors, who deal with people's lives, put in the effort to learn the (cognitive and non-cognitive) skills required?

B) Sharing 'tricks' or 'insider scoops' would be highly unethical and against our philosophy of what a "good doctor" is all about (more about the "good doctor" in the next chapter) and you should be immediately alarmed if a book or admissions company claims to be sharing 'insider' information.

C) We have a strict policy at BeMo to only help students who are genuinely interested to become a medical doctor.

How should you read this book?

In the introductory chapter to follow we will define a "good doctor", give you an overview of each chapter in this book, and discuss how to best utilize the information in this book to your advantage. It is important to note that there is a lot of information in this book, and if you try to do everything at once, it may seem overwhelming and discouraging. This is why, as we recommend in the introductory chapter, it is best that you first read this book for pleasure from cover to cover, and then take one or two points from one of the chapters and gradually start to implement our recommendations. Once each task is completed, come back to the book, take one or two tasks to implement and repeat this process until you have gone over the entire book. The key terms here are gradual progression and consistency, because "Rome was not built in one day". Think of your journey to medical school (and your career as a medical doctor) as a life-long marathon, and make sure you enjoy every step of the way.

To your success,

Your friends at BeMo

Introduction: The "good doctor"

The good doctor! It is a term that comes to mind when one considers the selection process of medical school candidates. Today, more than ever, medical schools are chronically under attack by grand economic forces imposed on them by large pharmaceutical corporations (and their lobbying groups) who seek to gain hegemonic dominance of the medical profession for their own economic interests, while simultaneously turning the medical profession into a subservient arm of the state, which as Foucault described, strives to complete the bio political dream of homogenization and normalization in our post-modern societies. Thus, it should come as no surprise that medical schools are constantly combating these forces by reviewing, refining, and revising their admissions processes. The hope is that they can select those individuals who will one day be called "the good doctor" in the fight against hegemony and in the resistance against the influence of external forces that seek to divert the "good doctor" from her path of professionalism, compassion, empathy, social responsibility, and most importantly advocacy. As Michel Foucault succinctly emphasized, "the first task of the doctor is ... political: the struggle against disease must begin with a war against bad government. Man will be totally and definitively cured only if he is first liberated..." The good doctor fights to this end.

What else can be said about the "good doctor"? Well, aside from having a strong sense of sociopolitical awareness and a desire to advocate on behalf of the voiceless, the "good doctor" is someone who embodies the true definition of practicing both the Art and the Science of medicine, while always keeping in mind that his/her first duty is to the well-being and care of his/her patients. The "good doctor", being whole-heartedly devoted to the notion of evidence-based practice and the process of life long learning, is not only knowledgeable and up-to-date with the latest scientific and technical advancements in the field, but is also someone who is on a continuous journey of self-improvement and self-actualization in order to enhance his/her non-cognitive skills and emotional intelligence: the "good doctor" realizes that it is these latter qualities that will serve them dutifully in their most difficult times.

The "good doctor" also holds him/herself to the outmost ethical standards not only for the wellbeing and care of his/her patients, but also his/her profession, and society as a whole. Having specialized knowledge, the "good doctor" vows to use this knowledge for good and to never intentionally harm those who seek his/her help in times of need. And although her devotion to the tenants of her profession will be tested time and time again, the "good doctor" continues to persevere in the fight against those forces that seek to destabilize his/her profession and cause harm to the health of societies that he/she solemnly serves and protects. This is the definition of the "good doctor"! A genuine and a modern day superhero whose sense of humanity drives her to have positive impact on the world around her.

It was with the above ideas in mind, and the definition of the "good doctor," that we have written this book. Our aim was not to simply put together a "how to" book on successfully gaining admission into a medical program (although this book successfully does that). Our primary goal in writing this book was to educate the future generation of physicians on those important qualities and characteristics that will enable them to have maximal impact on the world around them. Through this book we hope to be able to show the rationale behind the medical school admission process and help many of you devise an appropriate road map to your final destination, if your final aim is to become a modern day superhero. And we are also not holding back in this book. Rather, we are sharing the same information we share with our students in our high-end one-on-one training programs with enrolment fees as high as $20,000 per person, depending on the program.

So how should you go about reading this book? Where should you start?

Here's an overview:

First, there is a lot of material covered in this book, and it is all very important to your success. We recommend that you first read this book for pleasure from cover to cover. Once you have read everything once, then you can use this book as your go-to-guide and refer back to specific chapters, as required.

Chapter one, as its title implies (*The Hippocratic Oath*) exclusively deals with the rationale and history of modern medical school admissions processes. It is crucial to thoroughly read this initial chapter so that you have a strong understanding of the rationale behind the grueling process before you proceed to subsequent chapters. The second chapter, entitled "*Plans are nothing, planning is everything*", discusses the importance of starting your application well in advance of the actual application deadlines. In this chapter, we highlight the importance of starting to work on your application even years in advance so that you create the strongest application possible. A critical point missed by most students.

Chapter three, entitled *Application Components and Processes*, discusses the various application components that are currently used as admissions tools by various medical. In this chapter, we discuss the personal statement, the autobiographical/work/activity sketch, CASPer (briefly – more in depth analysis in chapter 6), and the interview (again, briefly as it is covered in detail in chapter 7), but more importantly, we discuss how to make these components stand out among the thousands of other applicants.

Chapter 4 is a brief exposé on the Medical College Aptitude Test (MCAT). This chapter provides a general overview for the MCAT and briefly discusses the science and social science sections. Chapter 5 will be an in depth discussion of the Critical Analysis and Reasoning Skills (CARS) section of the MCAT. In our experience, this is the section of the MCAT where a lot of students struggle with and so we outline our strategies, approach, and a general overview of how to ace tricky section.

Suspecting that the admissions tool, **C**omputer-based **A**ssessment for **S**ampling **Per**sonal Characteristics or CASPer, will be used by most medical schools across North America, until it is replaced by a more reliable assessment tool, we decided to devote the entirety of chapter 6 to this topic. A former CASPer evaluator at the birthplace of the test, McMaster University, authored this chapter. He spends a portion of this chapter discussing the format, structure and functional details of the test, while details about how the test is scored and how one can formulate strong and appropriate answers to CASPer scenarios is presented at latter stages of the chapter. After reading this informative chapter, you will be very familiar with this admissions tool and be prepared to ace the test once it is time to apply.

Once we have discussed all of the pre-interview admissions tools and processes, it will be time to introduce the final hurdle in the medical school admissions process, the dreaded interview. Chapter 7 (*Admission Interviews-Preparation Strategies & Winning Mindset*), written by a former admissions committee member and interview assessor, will not only introduce you to the various interview formats that are currently in place, but will also show you how to appropriately approach the various question types that are encountered during panel/ traditional interviews, MMIs, MPIs, and other interview formats.

Chapter 8 is devoted to non-traditional medical school applicants. This chapter is intended to provide insight for those candidates who come from non-traditional science undergraduate backgrounds or those who are older than the typical applicant. Essentially, this chapter is for anyone who is interested in applying to medical school, but does not fit the stereotypical mold of the "general" candidate pool. The author, herself a non-traditional applicant, who had spent years working in various other professional roles and settings, has composed this very informative chapter.

Chapter 9, entitled *Case Studies: Do as they say AND as they do*, is a unique and fun read that has been devised with the aid of a number of our admissions experts. They have, very graciously, provided a case study on themselves highlighting their journey to medical school and beyond. These cases are intended to inform, invigorate and inspire you, and help you appreciate the amount of time, energy, planning and resources that goes into becoming a successful medical student, and a physician. As you read their stories, continuously reflect back on previous chapters to appreciate how each of these successful candidates incorporated the ideas discussed throughout the book in their successful plan and path to medicine. Chapter 10, *BeMo's TOP 8 RULES for Getting into Med School,* will go into myths surrounding medical school and provide rules that will allow you to stand out and get in.

The final chapter of this book is a useful guide put together by our BeMo team of admissions experts. This guide will help you learn more about the application process and provide you with valuable tools to draw upon during your preparation and application to medical school. The links and resources provided in this chapter are intended to be used in conjunction with the ideas discussed by the various authors of the book.

After reading this book, you will not only have a better understanding of the rationale behind the medical school admission process and the various admissions tools that are currently being used to select appropriate candidates, but you will also understand what it takes to develop those very important qualities and skills that will allow you to become a modern day superhero in a society that is desperately in need of superheroes. Our aim is not to show you any loopholes or magic bullets that will facilitate your acceptance into a medical program, but rather show you what is required and expected of someone who wants to be tagged as "the good doctor." Our hope is that by reading this book you will strive toward becoming an excellent physician who is knowledgeable, compassionate, ethical, socially responsible, and most importantly, socio-politically willing to advocate on behalf of those who cannot advocate for themselves. The world is in need of good doctors: are you one of them?

CHAPTER I

The Hippocratic Oath

The admissions process is a diagnostic test of sorts. Doctors don't order tests unless there is a reason: they're trying to make a diagnosis. In the same way, every step of your application process is a test that helps admissions officers "diagnose" you as prepared and suited for the medical profession. And, just like our knowledge of disease and diagnostics has evolved over time, so too have medical admissions. Each new generation of doctors has gone through a very different battery of tests than the one prior.

The world's first medical school, Schola Medica Salernitana in southern Italy, was founded in the 9th century. It seems that admission was open to men and women who could afford the eight years of study, thus making the criteria mainly financial. The history of the school is interesting but doesn't contribute much to preparing a successful application today. For the purposes of admission to a contemporary medical school, the most salient points about Schola Medica Salernitana's history to know are thousands of individuals travelled extensively to seek care at the school and the institution published several reference guides on medical practice and how to respectfully treat patients and their families. **This is important to note because it means that medical training is based upon service to others and has always emphasized clinical acumen and bedside manner.**

Keeping this in mind, it's more relevant to have an understanding of how medical school admission requirements evolved over the past century in North America. Formalized medical training was pioneered by the

1

University of Pennsylvania when the institution opened the Perelman School of Medicine. As more institutions were founded, the basic principles established by the Schola Medica Salernitana – that of service to others and equal emphasis between technical and interpersonal skill – continued. Yet, admission criteria were largely based on an applicants' previous academic success. Medical schools wanted to train students who were keen and enthusiastic to become physicians and had the basic knowledge and cognitive skills to complete their course of study. A foundation in interpersonal skills and practical experience were to be gained during medical school.

A major milestone in medical school admissions came about with the introduction of standardized testing to the admissions process in the 1920s. This test evolved into the Medical Collage Admissions Test (MCAT) and began as a means of assessing academic readiness for medical school. At that time, attrition rates in North American institutions were as high as 50%. The high drop-out rate was thought to be due to admitting students who could not adapt to the workload and heightened expectations of medical training.

General academic requirements were raised in addition to standardized testing. Indeed, attrition rates continued to decline and remained very low throughout the past century.

What remained elusive, however, was a means to assess applicants' non-cognitive skills and personal characteristics. At various points throughout the 20th century, medical schools across North America began to require personal statements, reference letters, and summaries of extracurricular, service, and leadership activities. Additionally, coursework outside the sciences (even those areas not intuitively linked to medicine like the fine and liberal arts) is now valued for helping applicants further develop important cognitive skills that will serve them well in medical school. Yet, there seems to be more than scholastic prowess to overall success in medical school. Even with the emphasis on high academic standards and a holistic approach there was still no reliable way to predict how students would perform beyond their first few years of classroom training in clinical encounters.

Success in clinical encounters depends upon interpersonal skills as much as academic acumen. Another major milestone in the admissions process was the introduction of the Multiple-Mini Interview (MMI) in the early 2002 as a means of assessing each applicant's professional qualities. This format was developed at McMaster University in Hamilton, Ontario as an opportunity for interviewers to discuss ethics, problem-solving ability, teamwork skills, and professional attitudes and beliefs with applicants. In lieu of the traditional interview where an applicant would have a lengthy interview with one or a few assessors, in the MMI, an applicant rotates through several different interview stations and is evaluated at each individual interview station by a separate assessor. The content discussed at each interview station varies and facilitates applicants' discussions on real-world scenarios, similar to the type of encounters they would face in the upper years of medical school. The creators of the MMI claim that by spreading out evaluations among different assessors and different stations, it decreases interviewer bias and allows for a more objective evaluation of the applicant. This was (inconclusively) shown to have a much more accurate appraisal of an applicants' abilities and a higher predictive value on an applicants' performance in medical school. However, only those successful in the beginning stages of the application process are invited to interviews where this type of appraisal takes place. Thus, a similar format for assessing non-cognitive skills has been introduced earlier into the application process in the form of the Computer-based Assessment for Sampling Personal Characteristics (CASPer). In the most general terms, this is a computer based simulated MMI that is completed individually and submitted to reviewers. It is important to note however that both the MMI and CASPer have since turned into for-profit companies by the creators of the tests who have contributed the most to their claims of efficacy. As such, in our opinion, it is critical to emphasize that as future "good doctors" and scientists, you must view such claims with a grain of salt. The jury is still out until additional independent research is done to prove the efficacy of MMI and CASPer in selecting appropriate candidates. And more importantly, as a good scientist you will note that nothing in science is forever and everything by definition can be improved.

In summary, medical school admissions have evolved over time to provide a well-rounded insight into an applicant's academic suitability and professional qualities. In some ways, we haven't really come that far from the principles of Schola Medica Salernitana: serve others and equally balance proficiency in the technological and interpersonal skills. In addition to medical education, the practice of medicine is based on old traditions that existed even before Schola Medica Salernitana. The history of those seeking to diagnose and treat others' ailments can be documented in ancient times. For the purposes of admission to medical school in the modern day, you don't need to know much detail about the earliest details in medicine's history. However, it is important to have an understanding of the founding principles of medicine and the different types of skills that have always been expected of physicians. Specifically, it's useful to have a conceptual idea of the Hippocratic Oath and an understanding of the art and science of medicine. While the science of medicine has changed over hundreds of centuries, the values that doctors must uphold and the art of their practice has remained virtually unchanged.

The Hippocratic Oath was written by Hippocrates, the "Father of Modern Western Medicine" and his teachings were foundational in Schola Medica Salernitana and other schools. This is the oath that new physicians take, binding them to uphold ethical principles. Though certain elements may become confusing or controversial or when viewing the oath in current times, knowledge of the oath will help you understand the non-academic qualities that medical schools seek in their candidates. The core ethics that physicians were expected to practice in ancient Greece are the same principles physicians must uphold today. These are the qualities upon which medical schools base their admission processes.

"I swear by Apollo the physician, and Aesculapius the surgeon, likewise Hygeia and Panacea, and call all the gods and goddesses to witness, that I will observe and keep this underwritten oath, to the utmost of my power and judgment.

I will reverence my master who taught me the art. Equally with my parents, will I allow him things necessary for his support, and will consider his sons as brothers. I will teach them my art without reward or agreement; and I will impart all my acquirement, instructions, and whatever I know, to my master's children, as to my own; and likewise to all my pupils, who shall bind and tie themselves by a professional oath, but to none else.

With regard to healing the sick, I will devise and order for them the best diet, according to my judgment and means; and I will take care that they suffer no hurt or damage.

Nor shall any man's entreaty prevail upon me to administer poison to anyone; neither will I counsel any man to do so. Moreover, I will give no sort of medicine to any pregnant woman, with a view to destroy the child. Further, I will comport myself and use my knowledge in a godly manner. I will not cut for the stone, but will commit that affair entirely to the surgeons.

Whatsoever house I may enter, my visit shall be for the convenience and advantage of the patient; and I will willingly refrain from doing any injury or wrong from falsehood, and (in an especial manner) from acts of an amorous nature, whatever may be the rank of those who it may be my duty to cure, whether mistress or servant, bond or free.

Whatever, in the course of my practice, I may see or hear (even when not invited), whatever I may happen to obtain knowledge of, if it be not proper to repeat it, I will keep sacred and secret within my own breast. If I faithfully observe this oath, may I thrive and prosper in my fortune and profession, and live in the estimation of posterity; or on breach thereof, may the reverse be my fate!"

Again, a detailed understanding of the oath is not necessary. However, you can see that physicians have always been expected to be knowledgeable, skilled, hardworking, and dedicated, and use these qualities to benefit the patient. As well, physicians have always had to be altruistic, trustworthy, and responsible. Some of these qualities can be learned in medical school as you grow into your role as a physician. But more importantly, these are qualities inherent to you as a person and are developed through life experience. This is why medical schools want to get a well-rounded individualized assessment of applicants. They want to know what motivated you to pursue medicine and how you have tried to prepare yourself for the field personally and professionally.

Hippocrates may have referred to medicine as an art but it is now considered both an art and a science. In the simplest terms, the science of medicine refers to the knowledge and application of evidence-based medical data. Using blood pressure for example, the science of this includes knowing how blood pressure is generated, what the purpose of blood pressure is, what a "normal" blood pressure is, and what adverse effects of "abnormal" blood pressures are. Additionally, the science of medicine includes knowledge of critical appraisal skills to be able to look at medical literature such as randomized controlled trials, assess their validity, and apply them to each physician's individual practice. To be successful at the science of medicine in the future, you need to demonstrate previous academic success and provide evidence that you'll likely be able to complete a rigorous medical program and learn and master important medical concepts. Experiences that are helpful in demonstrating these competencies include research and having presentations and publications. More significantly, admissions officers review your grade point average (GPA) and MCAT scores.

On the other hand, you can think of the art of medicine as referring to bedside manners: building a trusting relationship with the patient so you can respectfully complete a thorough history and physical exam, clearly and compassionately communicating a diagnosis, prescribing a treatment plan that reflects the patient's wishes, and carefully performing appropriate procedures. This also includes being able to tolerate uncertainty, mitigate risks, and being an advocate for your patients when appropriate. For this, admissions officers will review your personal statement, references, activity sketch and interview score. Do not underestimate the significance and value of the art of medicine; indeed, as you might have noticed, most markings of the "good doctor" arise from a mastery of the art of medicine. Together, all the elements of your application will demonstrate whether or not you have adequately prepared yourself to become a medical student and if your personal value system and academic potential is suited for entry into a training program.

The best predictor of future performance is past performance. No one can predict how you will behave in medical school or the quality of physician that you will be, but a track record of academic success and personal growth is evidence that you'll likely be successful in medical school and beyond. Every element of the application is closely analyzed so that admissions officers have the best opportunity to envision you in the future as a medical student.

Each experience will be meaningful to each individual in different ways. However, broadly speaking, there are some generalities in the type of qualities that each component of your application will speak to; different aspects of your application illuminate different aspects of a potentially successful physician. There are also "hidden" requirements that are fulfilled by completing your application on time and in good order. The process can be tedious and time consuming as you progress through each stage. Yet, completing a good quality application shows you pay attention to detail and can manage your time effectively, follow directions, and communicate effectively. Let's now consider each of these application components in a bit more detail.

GPA: Medical school is a professional school and admissions officers want to know that you'll be a successful student. Your GPA is evaluated to see if you have a consistent record of academic success. Achieving and maintaining a high GPA shows that you have the cognitive skills to succeed at understanding the scientific concepts in medicine. Furthermore, academic success implies that you have the time management and organizational skills necessary to balance all your learning requirements in a rigorous course load.

MCAT: The MCAT is also used to assess your academic skills. A successful and strong MCAT score demonstrates that you studied and mastered basic concepts in the foundational sciences. The MCAT is also devised in a manner that allows you to apply these foundational concepts to the questions that you've been given while simultaneously using other cognitive skills, like comprehension and critical thinking skills; skills that are crucial to becoming a successful medical student.

Non-academic Activities sketch: Your activities outside of the classroom speak to your values system and the non-cognitive skills that you have developed in preparation for medicine. As already mentioned, technical abilities are not enough to meet the expectations of the patient and thus the sketch is used to assess how apt you are at being proficient in the art of medicine.

Community Service/Volunteer (non-medical): Volunteerism is an almost requisite experience for prospective applicants. Giving your time and talents to others without any repayment is the definition of altruism; one of the core principles of medicine. Volunteer experiences also demonstrate that you are able to identify a need or worthy cause and are invested in making a positive change. Applicants can volunteer for a variety of different causes in a multitude of ways to practice and develop other important non-cognitive qualities, but generally, volunteering also speaks to being willing to serve, interested in the needs of others, and a willingness to go above and beyond expectations.

Community Service/Volunteer (medical): Volunteering within the medical field demonstrates competencies similar to volunteering outside of clinical areas. More importantly, volunteering in a healthcare setting demonstrates that you have an interest in the profession and have taken it upon yourself to gain more awareness and develop skills that will be necessary in the future. It's important to have an understanding of: the patient experience, the roles and importance of other professionals, and the way in which your local healthcare system actually operates prior to admission, as you'll come to rely upon this knowledge later on in your training.

Employment (non-military): Almost everyone needs to work for a living and employment is a practical, real-world experience that helps applicants understand this reality. Few applicants are able to work full-time during their academic studies and generally only older or non-traditional applicants have been fully employed. However, even short exposure to the work force demonstrates trustworthiness (as in handling money), ability to work with others, and that you can be a good representative of a company or organization.

Employment (military): Working in the military is a very different type of employment. Few people will understand the reality of military service, but it should be generally understood that valuable skills and qualities are developed from the nature of the work environment. Military involvement speaks to being both a good leader and a good team player, knowing how to stay calm under pressure, having the ability to exercise extreme discipline and pay attention to detail.

Research/lab: Whether clinical-based in the sciences, or otherwise, admissions officers look for applicants' research experience because it is important to the medical profession. This is the era of evidence-based medicine, meaning that medical practice is based on quality research. Demonstrating the skills to carry out research strongly implies that you'll be able to contribute to the knowledge base of your future profession. Just as importantly, research experience helps applicants develop an ability to effectively evaluate evidence and determine which projects are of high enough quality to affect clinical practice.

Presentations/posters: Many successful research or academic projects will result in presentations and posters. Having made a presentation or poster shows that you have completed high quality work. As well, these experiences require you to speak about your project so they allow you to practice your professional communication skills, both orally and in written format. Just as research experience demonstrates that you will be able to perform research in the future, presentations demonstrate that you will be able to explain the implications to your colleagues and patients.

Publications: Publications and presentations are similar because only successful and impactful work is published. They demonstrate that you have performed research at a high level.

Teaching/tutoring: Teaching or tutoring experience is important because doctors take on a teaching/tutoring role in their careers. In fact, the word "doctor" comes from Latin meaning "to teach". This does not just refer to formally instructing medical students and residents, but counseling patients. For example, doctors will counsel their patients on a healthy lifestyle and preventative care, how to take their medications, post-operative care and so on. This requires communication skill and an ability to simplify complicated material to relevant details that a patient can comprehend. And this can be practiced in teaching and tutoring experiences.

Honors/awards/recognition: Any type of recognition stands out on applications because they allow admissions officers to infer certain qualities from your application. These are likely awarded based on your academic and non-academic record and receiving such an honor is a tangible proof of your abilities.

Conferences attended: Physicians will be responsible for maintaining their competencies and increasing and updating their knowledge base throughout their careers. Many physicians are able to do this through attending conferences. Having previously attended conferences as an undergraduate, shows that you take initiative and are self-directed in your own learning.

Intercollegiate athletics, artistic endeavors, extracurricular, hobbies, and avocations: Many applicants shy away from listing activities that seem less formative or are not intuitively linked to medicine. Medicine is a demanding profession and sustaining your enthusiasm throughout your career requires work-life balance, so admissions officers want to see your outside interests. Being involved in athletics in any form implies that you have an awareness of a healthy lifestyle and understand the importance of physical activity. Spending some of your time on artistic endeavors and other hobbies shows that you have invested your free time into activities that you enjoy, and that these activities can be used for stress management in the future. Activities you take part in on your own time personalize and round out your application.

Leadership (not listed elsewhere): Physicians are seen as leaders in healthcare and in their communities. In the future, you'll be tasked with being an effective leader on both the micro (as in within the healthcare team) and/or the macro (as in within broader community or healthcare system) scales. Therefore, leadership is an essential quality that will be assessed in all of your sketch entries even if you haven't listed an activity specifically in this category.

Personal Statement: Your personal statement lets admissions officers know your motivation for pursuing medicine and allows you to elaborate on how you prepared yourself for medical school and your career afterwards. You will be evaluated both on your suitability for medicine and how well you express these ideas in writing. Communication skills are an important competency for a physician and expressing yourself thoughtfully and clearly will facilitate your other skills and qualities. It is, therefore, important you describe relevant personal experiences and highlight a few of your most meaningful non-academic activities.

CASPer: Medical schools that require CASPer do so as another means of evaluating your non-cognitive and interpersonal skills. Because this is done under a time pressure with minimal time to prepare, it is claimed to allow for an honest insight into your judgment and personal ethics as well as your ability to think clearly and communicate effectively in stressful situations.

Interview: The interview is the only opportunity for medical schools to meet you in person prior to making their offer of admission. Regardless of how your interview is structured, you will be assessed on your communication skills, the content and quality of your response, and your suitability for the medical profession. For as comprehensive and detailed your paper application may be, there are some aspects of your personality/characteristics that just can't be evaluated unless meeting face-to-face. This includes your demeanor, ability to stay calm under pressure, clarity of language, ability to consider multiple perspectives before arriving at a decision, and diplomacy when making a point. The impression you make in person allows medical schools to envision how you would be face-to-face during a patient's appointment, meeting with colleagues, or in the public arena in the future.

Reference letters: Referees tell medical schools their impression of you as an applicant and speak to your personal character. Medical schools want this perspective because learning of how individuals you've worked with view you, is helpful in determining the impression you will make on your future patients and colleagues.

Our understanding and practice of medicine is in constant evolution and admission to medical training programs will continue to adapt to these changes. The requirements of applicants seem quite daunting and can be tedious and time consuming to complete. However, keep in mind by the time you are ready to apply for medical school, you have already done the hardest work: you have applied yourself in your academic program and MCAT preparation to achieve high marks and acquire a large body of knowledge, sought out rewarding extracurricular activities to foster personal growth, explored opportunities to expand your understanding and ability to contribute to an academic field through education and research opportunities, and developed an appreciation for the importance of self-care and balance by maintaining interests outside of medicine. Investing in these experiences and reflecting on what you learned will give you the ability to capably communicate why you wish to be a physician and demonstrate the personal and professional strengths you have to be an asset to your program and field. As well, developing strong and supportive relationships with colleagues and supervisors will demonstrate your abilities and allow others to speak on your behalf with strong references. Hopefully, expressing the strengths of the various components of your application will allow all the hard work to pay off with a successful admission to medical school!

References:

de Divitiis, E., Cappabianca, P., & de Devitiis, O. (2004). The "schola medical salernitana": the forerunner of the modern university medical schools. *Neurosurgery, 55(4),* p 722 – 744.

Eva, L., Reiter, H., Rosenfeld, J., & Norman, G. (2004). The ability of the Multiple Mini-Interview to predict pre-clerkship performance in medical school. *Academic Medicine, 79(10),* p 40-42.

Ludmerer, K. (2004). The development of American medical education from the turn of the century to the era of managed care. *Clinical Othopaedics and Related Research, 422,* p256-262.

McGaghie, W. (2002). Assessing readiness for medical education: Evolution of the medical college admissions test. *Journal of the American Medical Association, 288(9),* p1085 – 1090.

Sheridan Libraries and University Museums. (2015). Hippocratic Oath, Modern Version. *Retrieved from:* http://guides.library.jhu.edu/c.php?g=202502&p=1335759

CHAPTER II

"Plans are nothing, planning is everything."-Dwight D. Eisenhower

The primary goal of this chapter is to help you plan a successful path well in advance of your actual anticipated date of application. This chapter is all about meticulous planning and preparation and it's most appropriate for students in early undergraduate or late high school. Our goal is to teach you how to identify the essential qualities medical schools look for in their applicants so that you can "reverse engineer" your path. This chapter contains no shortcuts because the only way to gain experience is to get involved in appropriate non-academic (and academic) activities that convince the admissions committees that you have acquired those essential qualities. But when should you REALLY start thinking about your medical school applications?

The simplest answer to this question is "as soon as possible." However, it really isn't as simple as that. There is a lot of background information and context needed to know exactly when (and how) to begin applications for medical school. First, you should know the purpose of a medical school application. Applications are used to assess your readiness – professionally and personally - to enter medical school. You prove that you are academically prepared for medicine by demonstrating cognitive skills – academic ability - through your scholastic record (GPA and MCAT). You prove that you are professionally suited for medicine personally by demonstrating non-cognitive qualities: empathy, compassion, reliability, trustworthiness, hardworking, and so on. These can be demonstrated on your CV and activities sketch and personal statement. Your personal statement is also an opportunity to talk about your motivation for pursuing medicine and your interests and goals in medicine. It's not just restating your resume. Personal statements are your only opportunity to put your individual stamp on your application and let schools know more about you as a person and potential student and colleague.

First, you should determine what type of applicant you are. There are three broad categories:

A) Traditional applicants

"Traditional" refers to the applicant's undergraduate program and their age when applying to medicine. These are students who are applying to medicine while currently completing or having recently completed an undergraduate degree and are usually studying something science or health related, which they chose with the intention to pursue medicine.

B) Non-traditional applicants

"Non-traditional" most often refers to applicants who have chosen to study in something other than the "traditional" health or science program. For example, anthropology, engineering, or astronomy would be considered "non-traditional." These students may be applying at the same age as a traditional applicant or applying later as a mature applicant.

C) Mature applicants

"Mature" refers to an applicant's accumulated life experience at the time of application. Typically, these are older adults who have had a prior career or have begun a family instead of applying during undergraduate studies. Students who have completed a graduate program such as a Master's or PhD, are also considered mature applicants.

It's a myth that medical schools favor admitting traditional applicants. While a significant portion of medical students are traditional applicants, this more likely reflects that these students are the most inclined to pursue medicine instead of schools' preferences. Regardless of the type of applicant you are, the purpose of your application is the same and you will be required to demonstrate the same level of academic success and high degree of personal and professional qualities.

One of the best approaches in applying to medical school is to think of it the way an athlete approaches training. The most successful athletes are those that train for a long time and are highly developed in different ways, like strength, endurance and speed. Think of what you would do if you wanted to run a marathon. You would commit yourself to spending the necessary time training and making sure you do that over an appropriate length of time. You would make sure that you are not only a capable runner, but have power and flexibility as well. Keep this in mind as you learn more about your training for medical school.

In the most basic terms, academic suitability is demonstrated by achieving a high GPA and MCAT score. This shows that you can acquire knowledge and have the cognitive ability to practice medicine competently and accurately. You'll show you are personally suited for medicine by participating in diverse extra-curricular activities with a wide variety of roles and responsibilities. These activities will allow you to develop the attitudes and qualities necessary to practice medicine compassionately and ethically. You have to show that you are successful on both fronts; high achievement in school will not compensate for having poorly developed non-cognitive skills and vice-versa.

How to choose the best school and program of undergraduate studies

One of the biggest keys to academic success is using self-reflection to decide what you want to study. Recall that medical schools do not have a preference between traditional, non-traditional, and mature applicants. This means that you have the option of studying whatever program you want and can still be successful while applying to medicine. The only condition to this is that you complete the necessary pre-requisite courses and credits. Think long and hard about what you want to do. What are your strengths? What motivates you? What is important to you? What do you value? Just as importantly, reflect on what you do well and what program you think you can receive the highest marks. Also consider what program will allow you to dedicate time in pre-requisite courses and courses that are helpful for the MCAT.

Students perform best at the things they are passionate about. What are you most interested in? What fascinates you? Answering these questions will give you an idea of what undergraduate program is the best fit for you. You've probably already thought about what kind of person you are, what kind of work you want to do, and what kind of impact you want have on the world around you. And most likely you have already discovered that you're passionate about medicine. Use the same self-reflection to decide what course of study you're passionate about. Whether or not that's the sciences or arts, or a profession like engineering or teaching (or anything else). The most important thing is to choose what will make the most sense to you. When you're excited about what you're learning, you'll study harder and perform better and that goes a long way to achieving good grades. You'll probably also build stronger connections with your peers and professors and have a strong support network and more opportunities and resources moving forward. It will also make life in general a lot more enjoyable if you're doing what you like instead of what you think you "have" to do.

As challenging as it is to decide what to study, it can be equally difficult to decide where to study. Again, putting it simply, the best school to attend is the university that you feel is the best fit in the city where you want to live. This could be a small or a large school that is close to home or far away. But, as there were lots of things for you to consider when choosing your course of study, there are also lots of things to think about before deciding on a specific school. Many applicants mistakenly think that having a degree from an acclaimed school will help their application stand out. However, don't overlook smaller, lesser-known schools in favor of bigger names. **Keep in mind that where you went to school says much less about you than how you performed: it's a GPA requirement, not a school name requirement.** No one school offers an advantage over another. Very briefly: smaller schools may offer more opportunities to develop connections with peers and professors but fewer academic or extracurricular opportunities; larger schools, on the other hand, may be more competitive and professors may be more distant, but you will have more opportunities to be involved at school and in the community. All this is to say that deciding on a university is a personal choice and medical schools do not choose applicants based on where they did their undergraduate degree. The only thing that matters is your GPA. Remember that your goal is to develop a strong application and to gain successful admission to medical school. You will need to talk to students and alumni, inquire about research and extracurricular opportunities, and look where you can continue your hobbies and activities of interest. Don't choose a university based on name recognition or reputation. Choose instead where you feel you have the best opportunity to succeed and the most resources to have meaningful experiences.

When to write the MCAT?

Now, what about the MCAT? Well, similar to other items we've discussed above, there is both a simple answer and a practical answer to know when it is the best time to write the MCAT. **The simple answer is that you should write the MCAT when you feel 100% ready to write the MCAT. Period.** The practical answer is that you want to balance the timing of the exam with completing enough coursework or independent study to have the necessary background for the test, while still leaving time in your university career to re-write it if you perform poorly. Most traditional applicants will choose to write it after their second year of university as the bulk of the MCAT content is covered in lower year courses. Most non-traditional or mature applicants probably will choose to write it as soon as they can to not delay their application. While many schools will consider your most recent scores (i.e. giving you the option to re-write without it penalizing your application), the expense of time, energy, and money makes it worth writing only once. Also, don't let having the option of delaying or re-writing the MCAT distract you from making your best effort to prepare. **The most successful applicants are those who set out to write the exam only once, whenever that may be.**

Don't forget as well that your GPA and MCAT scores don't count for everything in your application. Think of it this way: **most patients don't want a doctor who is only a good diagnostician and prescriber; they want someone who listens and communicates well and is empathetic to their situation. A doctor they can trust.** While having high grades and a strong MCAT score gives medical schools an idea of how you would "treat" a patient, they don't tell them how you would "care" for a patient. It is only through non-academic activities that you develop the non-cognitive abilities that medical schools are looking for in future doctors.

Non-Academics

Just like self-reflection was helpful in choosing an academic path, it can be a useful tool when deciding which extracurricular activities to pursue. As mentioned above, there are no required programs of study and it is not advantageous to study at a particular school. Similarly, when it comes to non-academics there are no required extracurricular activities. Medical schools don't choose successful applicants based on a specific type of experience that they participated in as an undergraduate. Rather they want to make sure that you took part in specific non-academic activities because you were passionate about something. They want to make sure that you are well-rounded and have interests outside of your textbooks. They also care to see that you demonstrate commitment and progression over time, rather than jumping from one activity to another just to fill up your application. Ask yourself what kind of care would you like to provide future patients and what skills will you need to do this? What experiences offer you the opportunity to develop these skills? What kind of impact do you want to have on the people around you and how can you have a positive influence? Work for causes you believe in, engage in activities that you enjoy, and interact with people who inspire you. Because of your commitment to doing well in school you're going to be spending a lot of time studying so you want to make sure that you're devoting your time in areas where you're fulfilled. You'll find you enjoy yourself more, do a better job, and make a stronger impression on the people you will work with when you pursue your passions in non-academic activities. Even though you may be passionate about being a physician, you haven't yet had an opportunity to show what you can do as a physician. When you pursue activities that you're passionate about and perform well in, you tell medical schools that you'll likely accomplish your goals and succeed in medicine as well.

Clinical or medical experience is a little different from other types of experiences, however. **It is extremely important to have some type of clinical or medical experience prior to applying.** This can be volunteer, employment, or shadowing. Working with patients and doctors shows that you have an interest in medicine and this is paramount to a successful application. It just makes sense: why would you be applying for something that you knew nothing about? Further, you can share insights into the healthcare field that can be invaluable to strengthening your application. It's important to medical schools that their students understand the roles and responsibilities of a physician including the ethics they must use, the demands and stresses they face, and the actual reality of their job. It's also important that medical students understand challenges that patients face and have developed strategies to make the patient experience more positive. While most non-cognitive abilities can be developed in any experience, the perspective on the actual practice of medicine can only be gained through clinical or medical experience.

You will discuss your non-academic activities in an activities sketch, which is an important part of your application. It allows assessors to determine whether or not you have the life experience and skills and qualities necessary to become a medical student. The following is a guideline of what types of activities you may wish to include and what non-cognitive skills they may demonstrate. Even though some activities will demonstrate different things, this is a basic framework to use going forward. A helpful strategy is to first make a list of all your activities and come up with descriptions on your own. Then, visit the website of medical schools in which you're interested. Many of them will list their selection criteria including the skills and qualities they want to see in their applicants. If you believe any of their desired qualities were demonstrated in your own experience, make sure to say so!

The possible categories include artistic endeavors, community service (medical and non-medical), extracurricular activities, awards,

intercollegiate athletics, leadership, military service, paid employment, physician shadowing, research, and teaching.

These categories should cover every type of activity in which you participate. The few things that don't quite belong can go in an "other"
category and can demonstrate more or different qualities than the ones
you've listed. It's easy to spend time categorizing and labeling different
activities and switching these around. Having a strong activities sketch
is less about the category and title of each activity and more about how
you describe the activity and why it is important in your application. Of
course, activities have to belong in an appropriate and proper category,
but there's a lot of overlap between categories.

It's okay to pick one category out of the two or three where you think
an activity belongs. For example, you could include your volunteer tutor
position in either community service or tutoring as long as you described
it well. Think of it like ordering dinner at a restaurant. Sometimes an
appetizer sounds like it could be an entrée, but overall the menu seems
to make sense. The name of the meal gives you an idea of what you're
going to get. Still, you really only care about how the food tastes! How
the food tastes is analogous to how you describe your activities. You want
to give an assessor an idea of what you did in that activity but emphasize
the skills and qualities you developed. It's important to mention the
impact this experience had on you and your ability to make an impact
while doing this activity.

Case study

One applicant, Sarah, always found herself drawn to working with children. In high school, she had a regular babysitting job and joined fun-
draisers for the pediatric floor at her local hospital. When she started
university, Sarah realized how much she enjoyed being around kids and
how important advancing children's causes was to her. She found an
opportunity to help in a class with elementary school students and dedicated an hour a week throughout the school year volunteering for the
entire duration of her undergraduate studies. Her activity sketch might
look something like this:

Activity Type: Community Service/Volunteering – Non-medical/clinical
Name: Volunteer Teaching Assistant
Description: I worked with a schoolteacher to implement lesson plans for her elementary students and assisted individual students with their assignments. It was enjoyable finding creative ways to make learning fun. As well, I learned about the importance of respect, sensitive boundaries, and caring support when forming a relationship with children.

You can see from this example that Sarah emphasized what she gained from the activity, and highlighted some important non-cognitive abilities in communication and partnership. These skills would not have been developed as easily in a purely academic exercise. Even though it is not medically related, it is easy to picture Sarah forming a good rapport with a pediatric patient and being sensitive to his or her needs.

It may seem that the motivation to pursue extracurricular activities is simply to fill out your application. Sometimes applicants feel pressure to pad their resumes, meaning they participate in activities that "look good" as opposed to those that are enjoyable or rewarding. This is not the right mindset and, while it might lead to an impressive resume, you probably won't enjoy yourself or gain as much from experiences you would have if you pursued your interests. This is another reason why self-reflection is important. Think of what activities allow you to act on what you believe in and reflect your values. In this manner, you're more likely to actually develop the skills and qualities medical schools are looking for in their applicants. Don't forget that the application process is meant to prepare you for medicine. You need to participate in meaningful activities where you are enthusiastic about the tasks you take on in order to be ready and excited about the experiences and responsibilities you will face as a medical student.

It may also seem that the motivation to choose certain non-academic experiences is to have more items to add to your application. Again, sometimes applicants feel the need to participate in as many activities as possible. This is also not the right mindset and probably won't return any investment in your time. It's important to highlight another important factor that you will be evaluated on in your activity sketch. **Not only**

will you be evaluated on your maturity and growth in your activity, you'll also be assessed on your time commitment. Intuitively this makes sense. First, you're more likely to actually gain the skills and qualities you want to demonstrate the longer you're involved in an activity. Second, devoting a significant time commitment to an activity infers that you have a lot of other non-cognitive abilities, like commitment, dedication, and reliability. Third, spending more time in an activity gives you more opportunities to build support networks, find more opportunities to participate, and provides more connections with individuals who would be good choices for referees. **One of the most important things to remember when choosing activities is quality over quantity.**

To answer the question asked at the beginning of this chapter, the best time to begin planning for medical school really is as soon as you can. This is because it gives you the most amount of time to figure out the best fit for your choice of university and program of study, and the added time allows you to find non-academic activities that are valuable learning experiences for you. **The importance of planning early cannot be overstated. The most obvious reason for this is that developing the qualities necessary to be a good physician takes a long time so it requires a long-term commitment.** For several reasons, some applicants are not able to plan early and find either their academic or non-academic record or both, lacking. This doesn't mean that they are doomed. It does mean, however, that they need to begin self-reflection and thoughtful planning as soon as possible. It will take time to create a record of scholastic success and extracurricular involvement. Not planning early results in delays to applications; because application cycles occur annually, these delays can be years. You may have heard of applicants who are successfully admitted to medical school without actually having planned on attending or who chose to pursue medicine late. Because non-cognitive skills are transferable and can be obtained in different ways and the fact that medical schools have no preference for academic or experiential background, this only shows that it's possible to develop skills necessary for medicine without directly pursuing the field. It doesn't mean that you can be successful sending in an application on a whim. But a close look at those applicants would show they had a strong academic record and a diverse range of experiences. They would be able to apply these skills to any field and be successful, including medicine. Make sure you give yourself the best opportunity for success and begin planning early.

Planning early also gives you an opportunity to demonstrate a commitment and perseverance that can't be shown if you begin later. Moreover, planning early allows you to invest more time in your non-academic experiences. Since the purpose of your non-academic experiences are to acquire the professional skills and qualities of a physician, the benefits of planning early intuitively make sense. Medical schools will have more confidence in your development of non-cognitive abilities when you show that you have spent more time developing them. Think again about marathon runners. How likely is it that someone who only trained for a few weeks will cross the finish line? Now remember the example of Sarah, the applicant who volunteered in a schoolroom. How many skills could she have acquired in only a few days in that activity? How strong could her skills in working with children be after a month? Imagine that Sarah states that she was involved in that activity for an entire year. It's easy to believe that Sarah has developed excellent non-cognitive abilities in that time. It's also easy to see that she is dependable and trustworthy for having made a long-term commitment to an activity.

Committing yourself to opportunities also opens doors to new opportunities. The longer you stick with an activity, the more likely you'll be able to progress within it. An important quality to demonstrate is the ability to mature and grow and use your existing skills to acquire new ones. Sarah is a good example of this.

Activity Type: Community Service/Volunteering – Non-medical/clinical
Name: Volunteer Teaching Assistant
Description: I worked with a schoolteacher to implement lesson plans for her elementary students and assisted individual students with their assignments. It was enjoyable finding creative ways to make learning fun for children. As well, I learned about the importance of respect, sensitive boundaries, and caring support when forming a relationship with children. After one year in this position, I took on the role of trainer for other classroom volunteers and organized our schedule. I became effective at problem solving and time management. I also learned how best to balance the needs of individuals and the whole team in which I worked.

Sarah has been able to demonstrate additional valuable skills in this activity because of her progression. This would be the expectation of any medical student. For example, you might not even know how to properly take vital signs in your first year of medical school. But, by the end, you'll not only be expected to take vital signs, but interpret what they mean, provide any treatment necessary, and teach others to take them properly too. Sarah has shown she will likely be able to do this because she has demonstrated that she is capable of taking on new responsibilities and helping others make the same progression.

In addition to providing more opportunities, early planning helps you create more relationships that will be helpful in your application process. Many applicants wonder who will make a good reference and struggle to find a strong referee. If you make a long-term commitment to performing well in school and investing your time in meaningful activities, you will prevent a lot of this anxiety. The more time you spend in an endeavor the more time you give a potential referee to get to know you. This means he/she will be able to provide a more comprehensive and positive reference because he/she will have seen you in multiple roles and have observed your growth and progression in the task.

The better a reference knows you, the better he/she knows your motivation for medicine and is invested in your success. Early planning allows you to take the time to get to know your professors and score highly in their classes. You'll also be well positioned to take on scholarly activities and perform well. This will go a long way to getting a strong academic reference. Also, early planning allows you to make a connection with your co-workers and supervisors in non-academic activities. Not only can they attest to your skills acquisition, but they can describe your character and suitability for medicine in a far better way than if they did not know you for the same amount of time. This is extremely helpful in obtaining strong personal references.

In closing, like professional athletes, successful medical school applicants dedicate a lot of time to their training in advance. By making the same effort to decide on your best options for university, programs of study, and extracurricular activities, you'll not only cross the finish line but have a crowd cheering for you along the way.

CHAPTER III

Application Components and Processes

Each medical school prides itself on a different institutional culture, curriculum, and learning style. The aim, each year, is to attract the best and brightest of medical school applicants from across the world. At entry, some of these schools are interested in fostering research clinician careers. Some are devoted to the union of social science and medicine. And yet others are just trying to fill the gaps in their communities.

When selecting medical schools for your application, there are a number of essential criteria to consider. This chapter, along with providing you with information on the various application components involved in the application process, will also help you approach school selection with a clear framework for decision-making. We do not recommend that you apply to all of the schools in North America. It will be way too much work, money and confusion. Further, it will muddy your vision for what kind of doctor you're interested in becoming. Pay careful attention to the advice in the subsequent pages so that by the time you are finished reading this book, you have a clear sense of where you will apply and where you are likely to attend. Use the Application Tracker at the back of this chapter to keep track of your approach to filtering your selections. This is especially important for students applying to medical schools in the United States.

Application Procedures

There are three main portals in North America that serve as centralized application services for medical school applicants. The largest is AMCAS, the American Medical College Application Service (AMCAS), which is operated by the Association of American Medical Colleges (AAMC). Most US medical schools use AMCAS as their centralized application service. AMCAS is also one of the largest repositories of medical school admissions data in the world. Their reports and online information systems are especially valuable for anyone who plans to apply widely across North America and anyone interested in applying as a non-resident of either the US or Canada. See the Additional Reading at the end of this chapter for essential AMCAS resources.

The second portal is the Texas Medical & Dental Schools Application Service (TMDSAS) (https://www.tmdsas.com). This is the portal for all public medical, dental and veterinary schools in the state of Texas.

The third portal is the Ontario Medical School Application Services (OMSAS) (http://www.ouac.on.ca/omsas/). This is the portal for all six Ontario medical schools. Ontario has the highest number of medical schools of any province. Visit the main sites of each of these portals early in your application year to understand policies, procedures, fees and deadlines. Following the instructions well in advance of the deadlines will save you from being trapped in the intricacies of the online portals the night before your application is due.

For any medical school that does not participate in a centralized application portal, their admissions requirements and application procedures will be available directly on their websites. These include all applications outside of the province of Ontario and all those in the United States that use neither AMCAS nor TDSMAS.

Programs

The MD admissions process has been complicated in the past several decades by the emergence of joint programs reflecting the increasingly complex nature of healthcare, health system innovation and clinical research. Funding for joint programs is especially prevalent in the US.

Joint Program options available through AMCAS:

1. MD/Master of Business Administration (MBA)
2. MD/Doctor of Jurisprudence (JD)
3. MD/Doctor of Philosophy (PhD)
4. MD/Master of Public Health (MPH)
5. Summer Programs
6. Post baccalaureate
7. Baccalaureate/MD

Joint Program options available in Canada:

8. MD/Master of Business Administration (MBA)
9. MD/Doctor of Philosophy (PhD)
10. MD/Master's
11. Baccalaureate/MD

The Post Baccalaureate programs are typically one-year bridge programs to help disadvantaged or otherwise marginalized students gain entry into an MD program. They also exist to help non-science students prepare for entry to an MD program.

Baccalaureate/MD programs are seven-year programs where students gain entry into a combined undergraduate and undergraduate MD program from secondary school. These are slightly different than Early Acceptance Programs where students gain admission to an MD program after their first or second year of undergraduate studies by demonstrating remarkable academic potential.

Eligibility, Prerequisites & Criteria for Admission

The criteria for admission to each medical school in North America varies widely. This does not mean that gaining entry is easy. It is truly the difference between casting a wide and shallow net versus a narrow and deep net on the part of the institution. The choice of prerequisites is largely related to the mission statement of the medical school, and to the types of ideal candidates the school is interested in attracting.

Location

They say that the best medical school is the one that lets you in. For many who gain admission to medical school, the city is a second thought. You will go anywhere. It is important to be open to these kinds of opportunities. However, we also recognize that it's important to be close to family, if family ties are an important part of your life. If given the choice, we recommend a location that satisfies both your personal and professional lives. Having a relatively decent support network during medical school can make the difference between success and failure. It is a grueling time in your life and having access to the people that make you feel confident as a learner and as a person is very important. Don't underestimate your need for support.

The location also offers an important filter for your approach to applications, which is why we are beginning the discussion of selecting medical schools with location. The AMCAS system (MSAR) can be completely overwhelming when you first start to explore the portal. By narrowing down your approach to a geographical region, applying to medical school in the United States can be simplified. However, if your application has weaknesses, the more broadly you apply, the better your chances of admission. Location is one effective filter for selecting medical school to which you can apply but it doesn't work for everyone.

The universities also filter students by location. In Canada and the US, regional governments fund public universities in order to fulfill a training mandate of the next generation of healthcare providers. These providers make the state or province livable and constitute essential services. For this reason, these jurisdictions train small numbers of people who are residents from outside of that jurisdiction. This is especially true in Canada where international students can find it difficult to find a spot in medical school even if they are willing to pay the highest tuition prices. In the US, private medical schools typically accept applicants from all over the world provided they meet the eligibility requirements. There are several medical schools that treat Canadian students as Out-of-State applicants instead of international students.

A medical degree, no matter where you get it, will be a high-quality learning experience. But the cost of living in various cities, especially in America, is highly diverse. A medical degree in New York City will set you back upwards of $500,000 whereas a medical degree in Omaha, Nebraska will not. Consider your access to resources when making the decision about where to live.

Location also determines language of practice opportunities. If you are dead set on practicing medicine in Spanish, it is important to live in New Mexico, Texas, California or another state with a high concentration of Spanish speaking patients. The same is true in Canada if you're interested in practicing medicine in French. The Northern Ontario School of Medicine has plenty of opportunities for both Anglophone and Francophone medicine. But the most significant population of French patients will obviously be found in Québec.

If the school is close to your support system in a city that you enjoy with an effective transit, and if it offers good community participation and has a spirit of innovation, you will really feel good living in that city. If the school takes you across the country into weather that you're not familiar with and you're prone to loneliness and isolation, do yourself a favor and choose a different medical school. Medical school is stressful so the opportunities you have to step away from learning to enjoy the social aspects of life must be readily available and easily accessible in the city that you will be calling home. If you're very independent, consider that medical school could be one of those occasions where you may be more interested in finding a social niche given the demands of the curriculum and the experience of medical learning.

Academic Requirements

Grade Point Average
The Grade Point Average (GPA) is the best proxy variable available for scholarly aptitude. GPAs across North America are admittedly not terribly standardized. Medical schools realize this and use the MCAT and other measures of scholarship to assess applicants. Nevertheless, the GPA remains the bedrock of the academic requirements for admission to medical school in North America. The GPA number in isolation is important but so is the context. Most schools require full-time undergraduate studies

for between two and four years. They typically do not count the summer courses in the total GPA calculation. There are special exceptions made but these are the expectations you will have when you begin undergraduate studies. Additionally, most schools have prerequisite courses that must be reflected in your GPA. We will discuss these in the next section.

As you move through your undergraduate training, your grades must always be your first priority. Having a remarkable extra-curricular dossier with a stellar autobiographical sketch is necessary, but not sufficient, for gaining entry into medical school. Managing your time well is challenging but if you focus on achieving a high GPA above all else, your chances of acceptance will be increased. Additionally, if you change your mind about wanting to be a doctor at a later date, high grades always provide access to additional training opportunities and experience.

Achieving very high grades as an undergraduate requires planning and perseverance. Doctors are intelligent but they are not the most intelligent group of humans on the planet. Their intelligence is situated in essential character attributes – professionalism, discipline, commitment, resilience, lifelong learning, and willing to continuously self improve. If you can learn to adopt these characteristics as an undergraduate student, you will become a very good doctor.

GPA in the United States

The MD-granting institutions in the United States can be categorized in a multitude of ways: Private vs. public, whether they accept Out-of-State/International students, MCAT and GPA cutoffs, availability of Early Decision and Early Assurance Programs and many more. The most straightforward filter is location. However, if you have a weak academic record, location will not be a valuable filter for you. You should be willing to travel anywhere.

The US medical school with the lowest 10-90th Percentile GPA range is Howard University College of Medicine, a private college in Washington, DC. The GPA range of accepted applicants is 2.90 to 3.91. This means that 90% of accepted applicants had a GPA higher than 2.90 and also that 90% of accepted applicants had a GPA lower than 3.91. On the other end of the spectrum, Johns Hopkins University, a private university in Baltimore, Maryland, and Harvard University – maybe you've heard of this private university in Boston – both share the highest 10-90th Percentile GPA range of all the AMCAS schools: 3.72 to 4.0. The AMCAS portal remains your best resource for investigating the GPA requirements of over one hundred more American medical schools. Further, the AAMC's Medical School Admissions Requirements (MSAR) (https://www.aamc.org/students/applying/requirements/msar/) portal, which has a small annual fee, will provide each school's median GPA and MCAT performance for the preceding academic year as well as the national median for those scores.

To calculate your AMCAS GPA, use BeMo's AMCAS GPA Conversion Calculator (https://bemoacademicconsulting.com/amcas-gpa-conversion-calculator), or simply visit the official website of AMCAS.

GPA in Canada

Most universities in Canada have GPA cutoffs below which they will not consider your application. These minimums change annually and previous minimums shouldn't be used to predict future minimums. The vast majority of accepted applicants will have GPAs at the higher end and few applicants very close to the cut-offs will actually earn a spot. Individual websites for each medical school have the GPA profiles for accepted applicants (average accepted GPA) as well as the cut offs and you should focus on the average accepted GPA rather than any minimum cutoffs. Additionally, the Association of Faculties of Medicine of Canada publishes an annual admissions report.

The importance of understanding how your GPA maps onto a 4.0 scale, which is the scale used by OMSAS in Ontario, or percentage scores, which is used by many non-Ontario medical schools, cannot be overestimated. This is the first step to determining eligibility. An A+ is a 12.0 on McMaster's 12-point scale, a 90 to 100% on the University of Toronto's scale and an A on McGill's letter grading scale. These inconsistencies exist all over the continent. At the highest end of the scale, these differences aren't very relevant. However, in the middle of the scale, these grades have the ability to sink your GPA. For example, an 85% mark from the University of Toronto converts to a 3.9 on the OMSAS GPA scale. But an 84% mark converts to a 3.7 on the OMSAS scale. An 80% mark converts to a 3.7 on the OMSAS scale but a 79% converts to a 3.3.

Very quickly, you can start to see how the difference between an 84% and an 85% is very material to your overall academic picture. The even bigger difference lies in the discrepancy between a 79% and an 80%. One or more 3.3 entries on your Post-Secondary Institution Transcript can quickly slash the pool of schools to which you are eligible to apply, regardless of your MCAT scores.

GPA in Ontario

The Ontario Medical School Application Service requires direct entry of grades by the applicant into the application service. Then, OMSAS cross-references the entered grades with the official transcripts received. Transcripts that must be submitted for application to medical school in Ontario include all universities, colleges, CEGEP, junior colleges, graduate schools or other postsecondary institutions where you're registered presently or in the past. This includes exchange programs, transfer credits and work taken on Letter of Permission. This includes any postsecondary institution (university, college or CEGEP) at which you have registered, even if you have not attained a grade because a course is in progress, you withdrew or cancelled the course. This also includes institutions where you only took a summer course and these should be entered as Supplemental. These courses will be used to calculate your GPA at some schools and not at others. It is fraudulent not to include all transcripts that meet the criteria.

Transcripts from institutions in Ontario must be ordered from within OMSAS and those from outside of Ontario need to be ordered by the applicant to be sent from the institution to OMSAS in a sealed envelope. Prepare these submissions far ahead of the early October deadline. The final due date changes every year but OMSAS is prepared to accept transcripts between August 1 and the October deadline annually. Ensure that you have entered the institution in the section of OMSAS entitled "Post-Secondary Education" so that OMSAS knows to pair that transcript with your application.

OMSAS uses its own GPA conversion tool to standardize grades from all institutions across North America and beyond onto a 4.0-point scale. The BeMo OMSAS GPA Calculator is available for free online and you can use this to estimate your OMSAS GPA (http://bemoacademicconsulting.

com/OMSAS-GPA-Conversion-Calculator.html). You can also use the table provided by OMSAS.

Medical College Admissions Test (MCAT)

The MCAT is a standardized, multiple-choice examination designed to assess certain characteristics of medical school applicants and we will talk more about MCAT preparation strategies in Chapter IV and about the CARS section in particular in Chapter V. The test is administered by the AAMC (https://www.aamc.org/students/applying/mcat/about/). Medical schools around the world can choose to use the MCAT exam as a prerequisite for admission. Most medical schools find that it is a simple way to standardize assessment of academic acumen of the applicants.

Minimum MCAT scores can be set both by category and by total score. This is at the discretion of each university. Often, schools will select both a total score cut-off and a cut-off in each section as the basic MCAT eligibility criteria. A 2005 study by Julian examined the validity of MCAT performance for predicting success in medical school. He found that MCAT scores are a much more reliable predictor of medical school success than undergraduate GPAs, although the results have not be conclusive. Schools will also sometimes require that the MCAT be written in the previous five years so keep track of your AAMC ID and your test date so you aren't behind an entire application cycle due to an out-of-date MCAT scores.

While most schools do require the MCAT scores to be submitted with your application, not every school treats the MCAT in the same way. Some schools place little importance on the test in their evaluation of your candidacy even though they require that you take it. Some schools require that you meet certain cut-off scores in certain sections. For the most up to date information we recommend that you visit each school's official admissions website, as they regularly update their policies without notice.

Course Prerequisites

Course prerequisites vary from none to dozens of credits. This is why planning your course calendar as a first year undergraduate for the subsequent four years is essential. You need to be sure you get a spot in all of the required courses so that you can execute your undergraduate calendar at a pace that works for you.

At each institution, these courses will have a unique code. It is your job to be sure that the code of the course you took at your undergraduate institution fulfills the requirement at the medical school to which you are applying. Often, medical school websites will have guidance on whether or not your course counts towards the prerequisite. Every year, there is a lot of uncertainty around this topic so feel free to clarify with an admissions officer at the medical schools of your choice. They have the most experience answering these technical queries and have likely met students in your situation in prior application cycles.

Nonacademic Requirements

Alongside the MCAT's expansion into behavior and the bio-psycho-social model of illness, there has been a similarly capacious change afoot in medical school admissions. The medical school application process favors people who have had the time and money to participate in a large variety of research, volunteer and clinical opportunities. It also favors those with connections to the medical system not through nepotism or favoritism but just through early exposure to the language and epistemology of medicine. The people who are accepted into medical school currently are smart, dedicated and committed. But more often that not, they have a class-based "leg up". This is changing, but not very quickly.

If you don't come from this kind of privileged background, this does not mean you should give up. It just means that you'll have to work harder and pay closer attention than many of your peers. This is unfair but it represents a realistic approach to the process of applying to medical school in North America. You may have to work a full-time job in university while many of your classmates find volunteer positions in prestigious labs. You may have to start out volunteering in a lab and also working at a different job – in retail or waiting tables - until your performance in the lab is so impressive that they offer you a job. You may have to complete a Masters degree in order to have the funding and the flexibility to take the time to write your MCAT. You may have to self-study for the MCAT as opposed to taking a preparatory course. You may apply several times before gaining acceptance in medical school (even if you are a traditional applicant in the sense that you have a science background) so that you can learn the nuances of how doctors are expected to communicate with each other.

These expectations are not apparent to people who do not know any doctors or academics. This is one of the most understated reasons why disadvantaged, or even lower middle class, applicants are usually unsuccessful. If this is the case for you, we encourage you to invest in yourself and seek BeMo's help to groom you and your application in the intricacies of the application process. This way you will not be at any disadvantage. Also a word about finances again. Your journey to medical school, while in medical school, and beyond will be very expensive, but the long-term rewards vastly outweigh the short-term expenses. Therefore, if you are serious about getting into medical school, we recommend that you do whatever you can to invest in yourself, even if it means securing loans to pay for your undergraduate education, MCAT prep, application prep, CASPer prep, and interview prep. This is not something you want to skimp on, because if you do not get it right the first time, you will have to spend way more time, energy, and heartache redoing the application process.

Personal Statements

Medical schools ask for personal statements because they serve as a window into your personal story, your written communication skills and your connection with the human experience. They can also serve as a reservoir for your 'red flags', such as dubious ethical decisions, lack of self-awareness, unprofessionalism, or simply poor communications skills. Schools use the statements to figure out if they would look forward to seeing you every day in clinic because you're a hard worker without an ego, you're dedicated to learning, you can independently solve problems and you care about helping people.

We use the term 'personal statement' to cover any longer form prose required during the application. This includes brief personal essays where you are asked to answer a specific question and more general statements as well, such as the AMCAS Personal Comments essay. The guidance also applies to entries in the Autobiographical Sketch or Work and Activities Summary where you are asked to expand on a particular entry to share why it was most meaningful to you or how this entry shaped your path to medicine. Our advice stands for all of these writing forms.

AMCAS Personal Comments Essay

The AMCAS Personal Comments essay is a 5300-character essay, including spaces. For people applying to the MD/PhD programs, there are two additional essays to complete. Recall that, you are writing the same essay for every school to which you are applying through AMCAS. The essay is weighted differently at different schools.

AMCAS asks that you answer the following questions in the Application Instruction Manual:

- *Why have you selected the field of medicine?*
- *What motivates you to learn more about medicine?*
- *What do you want medical schools to know about you that hasn't been disclosed in other sections of the application? (i.e. Hardships, Challenges, Obstacles, Explanation of fluctuation in academic record).*

AMCAS Work/Activity Section

This is where you are asked to include all past experiences that you believe are relevant to your application to medical school

AMCAS Secondary Essays

Each medical school normally sends additional essay prompts to applicants after receiving their primary applications. These questions are unique to each medical school and are designed to determine whether or not the applicant fits well with the unique mission statement of each school.

OMSAS Essays/Questions

There is no overarching OMSAS single essay, as there is with AMCAS. Under each school's submission, schools can choose to ask you to write supplementary essays about certain topics.

Individual Schools

There is typically an essay component required in the application to most non-Ontario schools in Canada and most US schools that do not participate in AMCAS.

Personal statements are a careful dance between ensuring that you check all the boxes required by an admissions reviewer and tightly crafting a narrative about your life. We believe there are 11 essential characteristics of a strong personal statement. If you can be sure that your personal statements possess these characteristics, your statement will be well taken by most admissions committees.

Your personal statement must:

1. Be True and Be Yours

It is an act of professional misconduct to lie on your application to medical schools. This is not a great way to start your career. These false statements are difficult to catch but it does happen. Additionally, your statement will sound inauthentic. Personal statements are excellent training for interviews and if your personal statement is not true your interview responses will sound similarly inauthentic.

If you feel as though your life hasn't been interesting enough to stand out on a personal statement, you haven't thought about it long enough. This is a reason to brainstorm your statement excessively before you begin to write. Lurking in your life, somewhere, will be a valuable hook or frame for your statement.

Use the image on the subsequent page to help map pivotal moments in your life and then start to freely brainstorm about the meaning of those experiences. For example, maybe you have always found calculus very difficult. Your approach to dealing with your calculus problem has been to work harder than everyone else, own your vulnerability, seek out all of the extra training you can find and take additional courses just to improve your understanding of the subject. This is a pivotal moment that tells the reviewer so much about who you are even if you've not experienced very much hardship or strife in your life.

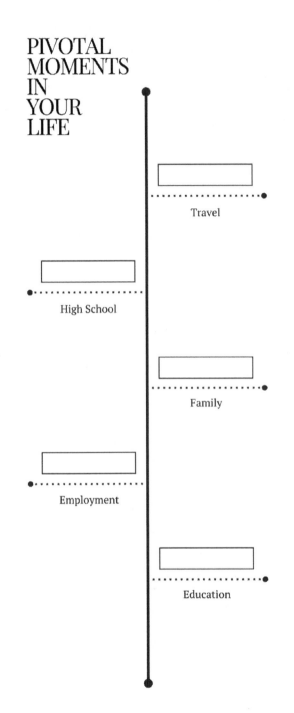

PIVOTAL MOMENTS IN YOUR LIFE

Travel

High School

Family

Employment

Education

2. Explain why you want to be a doctor

Personal statements often start by explaining why medicine is awesome. It is awesome, of course. But the admission committees already know that. You should explain why **you** want a career in medicine. What about the practice of medicine works with who you are? Naturally, this takes a lot of reflection around whom, exactly, you are. Start journaling or exercising some other creative muscle many months before the application – and ideally during the earlier half of the undergraduate degree – so that there is a coherent logic around why you want to be a doctor. And then communicate that as tightly and effectively as possible in your personal statement. Even questions that don't ask why you want to be a doctor should be connected in some way to this coherent logic.

For example, in a previous application cycle, the University of Toronto requested that all applicants answer the question, "Man is by nature a political animal" – Aristotle. Discuss what this quote means to you in regard to advocacy by physicians" in their brief personal essays. This question is asking you to do three things:

- *Show that you can follow instructions and provide some brief interpretation of Aristotle's statement. Because this statement is thousands of years old and has been the subject of thousands of philosophy doctorate degrees, the University of Toronto is not asking you to develop a new, original treatise on Aristotle's premise.*
- *Tell a story about a time where you used your communication skills to advocate on someone else's behalf, on your behalf or on that of the family.*
- *Link this story to an ethos that you carry around how physicians should behave. This allows the reviewers to picture you as a clinician, tactfully and creatively helping your patients get their needs met in a timely and effective manner, while also advocating within a larger sociopolitical health system context.*

I realize this sounds difficult. It is, especially if you are lacking in the social sciences department. This is why you must begin early when preparing for your personal statements. And you must diversify your education early on and take non-science courses.

3. Answer the question that they actually asked

If the question requires you to describe a conflict or challenge, make sure you actually do this. The AMCAS Personal Comments essays do not explicitly ask for this but if you believe that talking about a challenge you've experienced is part of your explanation for being a doctor, feel free to include a good description.

4. Use a narrative to paint a picture of who you are as a person

One of the best ways to illustrate that you've got the qualities required for medicine is by telling the admissions committees a story about your life. If you've worked through professional challenges, explain how you've done that and what you've learned about yourself. If you've demonstrated great perseverance, explain when and how. Remember that these stories must be true, yours and connected to why you want to be a doctor. These stories cannot effectively serve this purpose unless you've put a lot of effort into planning your statements in advance.

5. Address your core values, principles and ethical acumen

The story you choose to tell should also highlight one or two of your most tightly held values, principles or ethical positions in a logical way. If you are someone who is committed to community service, and have a track record of such service, your story should feature this and provide insight into why you care about your community. Saying "I value community service" when you've never volunteered a day in your life is absurd. Saying "My family is one where we support each other through challenge and loss," if this is true, is excellent because it lays the groundwork for telling a story, shows that you have a positive orientation towards close relationships and that you are principled.

6. Demonstrate the traits of professionalism

Professionalism is, at its root, about respect for the experience of others on your team or in your workplace. Stories or examples of when you have demonstrated respect in a workplace have real value, as long as you are connecting it to why you want to be a physician.

7. Establish your written communication skills

The ability to communicate a complex idea in a short space is among the most important of a physician's skills. Doctors communicate with each other and with patients using clear language without fancy or vague words. If you can demonstrate that you've already got this skill down pat with non-medical language, you will place yourself ahead of the pack.

8. Use clear and accessible language

Describing a clinical condition to a patient requires using specific but clear words. This is why your personal statement should do the same thing. Using large words in unwieldy ways makes you sound like you are compensating for poor communication skills. Use words that you believe most people understand. Read your personal statement back to a 14 year-old and then again to someone for whom English is not their first language to see if you're off the mark. Fancy words do not make you a good communicator. Listening and ensuring comprehension makes you a good communicator.

9. Be grammatically immaculate

If you give yourself several weeks -sometimes months- to write your statement, the chances of grammatical errors will decrease. Use the grammar checker on your word processor. Use the eyes and ears of other people to check and double-check. Read your statement out loud to yourself and I can almost guarantee that you will find an error. Use fresh eyes on your statement several times before you actually submit and you should be in the clear. We left a common grammatical error in this paragraph on purpose, can you spot it?

10 Possess flow, or readability

If the statement is pleasant to read, it will get read with more attention and appreciation. Flow is easier to craft through a narrative, which is why you should root the statement in a story that demonstrates characteristics one through five in this list. Flow takes time to build, which is why your statement should be etched out through many drafts and should also be based on an outline. That is, you should brainstorm, then outline, then draft and re-draft, then bring in editors and listeners. Then check and double-check.

11. Take only the most calculated of language and writing risks

Some applicants will have degrees for which they've written hundreds of thousands of words and read millions of words. These applicants should feel welcomed to take strategic, creative risks with their narratives but every point on this list still counts. Just because you know how to master a two-dollar word doesn't mean it belongs in your medical school application. Your personal statement should also maintain its concreteness – and be wary of the very abstract – while you take your creative risks. Just because you're a strong writer doesn't mean you don't need an editor. J.K. Rowling has an editor. Everyone needs an editor. You need an editor.

12. Address gaps in GPA, MCAT or other history as per the directives on the school's application guidelines

American medical schools through the AMCAS Personal Comments Essay ask candidates to explain gaps in the academic portion of their application in the personal statement. The same is true for several Canadian schools. Review the directions with a great degree of focus so that you leave no questions unanswered. The personal statement is the best place to address the concept of "distance travelled" in your application. We will explain this concept further in the coming pages but addressing vulnerabilities in a logical way could turn your weaknesses into attractive strengths.

This is true for the calculus example discussed earlier in this section. It's also true for life experiences like teenage parenting, multiple changes in academic course, lower grades and disabilities.

Red Flags

There are several commonly made, but entirely avoidable errors that you must NOT make on your personal statements. Before you submit your final draft, critically review your statement to ensure that you **do not**:

- *Re-list your entire CV or activity sketch. We can guarantee you will not be able to answer the question if your entire goal is repetitive self-promotion.*
- *Be pretentious. Every applicant is extraordinary, and so are you. Use your story to imply your excellence; don't hit people over the head with it.*
- *Criticize other applicants. This is unprofessional.*
- *Use very fancy words to make up for insecurities around writing skills. This is confusing.*
- *Ramble. This shows you submitted at the last minute.*
- *Rely on clichés. This shows you don't read widely.*
- *Describe a time you met a disadvantaged person briefly and use this as a rationale for why you want to be a doctor. This demonstrates a lack of self-awareness and limited understanding of the social determinants of health.*
- *Cast you as a victim. Even if you've been through terrible things, like escaping persecution or violence, the victim narrative is not one that will convince medical schools of your capacity. Cast yourself as an agent in your own life. This is a chance to explain your "distance travelled."*
- *Violate the character count. This is lazy. On most of the automated portals, this is impossible but it remains a concern on individual school applications.*
- *Simply listing adjectives. If you are simply listing some adjectives about yourself you are just going to sound arrogant at best. The best way to demonstrate certain qualities is to show them through past experiences and let the admissions committee choose the appropriate adjectives themselves.*

Autobiographical Sketches

Autobiographical sketches are like tabular stories about who you are. They break up your experiences in life into morsels and categories that make it easy to compare you, and your life, to the next applicant as fairly and clearly as possible. The sketch shares a technical, standardized portrait of who you are with the schools. The sketch takes a lot of time to build properly so start early. We always recommend that students keep a running list of what they've done, with whom and for whom over the years, starting at age 16. Sketches are required by AMCAS, TMDSAS, OMSAS and often the individual applications.

The best experiences for your sketches are:

- Longitudinal (over 12+ months)
- Show reach and variety
- Regular (i.e. four hours every week versus one day every eight weeks)
- Distinguished, or elite.
- Demonstrate progressive commitment
- Feature you in a leadership role
- Collaborative

Portfolio

As you are moving through your premedical years, you should start to build your portfolio. This can simply be a file folder in your hard drive with sub-categories for each activity, accomplishment, job, award or certification. Keep track of documents and correspondence this way. Additionally, at the completion of every activity, ask a leader – someone who will potentially become a verifier of that activity – if they wouldn't mind writing a letter or email with a few paragraphs about your role, the activities you performed and your special qualities. Your request should change in formality depending on whom you are asking. If you are writing to a Principal Investigator with which you've had a formal relationship, then speak more formally but still warmly.

Here is a template that you can use to request this letter (of course modify it into your own words!):

Dear [Name],
I wanted to write to let you know how important [the experience, activity, accomplishment] was to me as I move through my training. I benefited from [experience] in that I [list 1-2 items you learned or see differently now].

*I am writing to ask if you would be interested in putting together a brief
letter that I could use as part of my portfolio. As you know, my professional goals include becoming a doctor. I want to be a doctor because
[reason that is connected to the activity or experience]. Having a letter
from you that describes what I've done during [this experience], my role
and perhaps also some key strengths that I bring to [this experience] will
really help when it comes time to writing my application.*
*I am happy to provide whatever support I can with this. I really appreci-
ate it. I hope we can continue to be in touch.*
Thanks again.

[Name]
[Email/ Phone #]

Collect these letters and refer back to them when writing about your
story, strengths and accomplishments, as well as your areas of weakness.

Framing the Sketch

If there were some obvious framework to guide your pre-application
extra-curricular and academic lives, would you use it? Fortunately,
the American Association of Medical Colleges (AAMC) has developed several required core competencies for medical students and
future medical doctors and they can be found on the AAMC's website. Royal College of Physicians and Surgeons of Canada has also
developed such a framework – known as CanMEDS – to "describe the
knowledge, skills and abilities that specialist physicians need for better patient outcomes." These were not developed to show you how
to plan your life for medical school but it does help you see why and
how medical schools demand certain competencies and skills from
their learners.

Try to fit every piece of your past experiences into one of the following six areas. Even activities like school sports programs and dance
lessons fit if you plan your descriptions carefully:

Professionalism

Professionalism is an attribute that can be illustrated in a number of different ways. Work experience in any field is an excellent start. If you are coming from another career, that's an advantage to demonstrate professionalism. The actual area of work matters less than showing you've worked in teams or in a service role. Employment in a lab, research institute or clinic is also nice to have. Your reference letters should reflect your punctuality, your respect for others and for rules, as well as your general behavior.

Medicine is a self-regulated profession so having work experience that demonstrates use of ethical principles and high standards is a home-run in this category. Additionally, experience that shows commitment to excellence and high performance standards is reassuring to any admissions committee if the rest of the application is sound. Extra-curricular activities that show you are a committed, tenacious person who can foster a sense of camaraderie with many different kinds of people is valuable.

Communicator

This domain is dedicated to describing people who can handle tough situations with poise and clarity. Your personal statements go a long way in demonstrating communication skills, especially if you describe situations that involve conflict, errors and vulnerabilities. In describing these situations, make sure you dive into how your communication skills enriched and moved the situation forward. Ensure that you position yourself as an actor in those situations, not just a bystander.

Verbal communication skills will be highlighted in the admissions process and throughout your life as a physician. The ability to think quickly, adapt and be flexible during tense times with a patient is the basis of the 'art of medicine.' You can demonstrate these through participation in teams and group leadership. By volunteering in clinical settings and engaging in civil society, you can also show and improve your verbal communication skills.

Lastly, try to narrow down experiences that allow you to engage, reflect on and demonstrate empathy with other human beings. This is very different than pity and the distinction is key. If, in your personal statement, you talk about your two-week trip to Ghana and describe it in terms that express pity, rather than empathy, then your statement will not be achieving the goal. You must go deeper when describing these experiences and reflect on the inner changes that occur in the face of difficult situations. Empathy is one of the most powerful motivators, day to day, for physicians and empathy should inspire you to do your best. If you struggle to identify with the struggles and experiences of others, medicine will be a very difficult and complicated road.

Collaborator

A collaborator is someone who supports a team-based approach to health-care through his or her actions, thoughts and words. Extra-curricular activities that involve groups, teams and partnerships are best. Some research experiences work well in this domain and some do not. Labs that foster critical thinking and reciprocity are good fodder for discussing collaboration. Qualitative research also works well here because the subjects are, typically, human and your interaction with them is the basis of the research design.

Also, as with professionalism and communication, work experience in teams or in a service profession are very helpful. Don't be afraid to include experience serving tables or working retail, as long as you did so for over at least six months, and preferably 12.

Manager

The Manager domain is one of the most 'big picture' domains. It requires that you be able to zoom out from the individual level to a broader meso- or macro- system level. Later career doctors involved in health system administration make use of the Manager competency in an obvious way but so do doctors working exclusively in clinical settings.

You can demonstrate managerial competencies without experience as a manager. Activities that show good time management, skilled triaging of commitments, an awareness of scarcity of resources and time, capacity for creative problem solving under stress and acknowledgement of limitations are ideal. Just getting a university degree while also being involved in your community can show managerial potential. Leadership roles, however, are best for demonstrating the Manager competency. If you can articulate a leadership role wherein you improved the effectiveness of a team in a measurable way, this is ideal. Ideally, you can demonstrate increased commitment and leadership in one organization over time.

Health Advocate

This domain is about a physician's higher order duties to the community of patients and people they serve. Engagement in social justice or civil society work is the place to begin. You may also add clinical or research experiences around access to care, health inequities or the social determinants of health. Taking a course or more in health studies or health policy, with an eye towards vulnerable populations shows legitimate interest in health advocacy. Taking on volunteer opportunities with older adults, differently-abled people or people experiencing poverty is a good way to show your budding capacity as an advocate, if that work has meaning for you.

Personal narratives of marginalization that are insightful can also be very valuable here, provided that they are true and focused. The goal of sharing your experience of marginalization is to show that you recognize the various ways in which society and sickness interact, through power imbalances and discrimination. Additionally, when sharing global health experiences, the focus of your description should be on the meaning of the experience for you. Going to a low-income nation and writing in your personal statement, "We went and built a school, and life was better for the people in the village" doesn't communicate meaning nor that you understand the broader determinants of community wellness. An appropriate statement about a global health experience might discuss your own feelings, how it changed you, your attitudes, beliefs and skills.

Scholar

Your GPA is one place to start to demonstrate scholarship excellence. But the scholarship domain is also about "reflective learning" which requires self-awareness in the application, sharing and iteration of technical medical knowledge. Your GPA shows that you have technical knowledge but does not make it obvious how you engage with that knowledge.

The best way to demonstrate self-awareness in scholarship is to take courses from a variety of disciplines and to do very well in these courses. A chemistry student should take an English class. This shows academic bravery and insight into the need to expand how you learn.

Another way to demonstrate scholarship is through curiosity about the world. Travel, if possible, or take language lessons. Don't be afraid to try something outside of your natural aptitudes because this is the only way to develop new aptitudes. In your medical career, you will find new skills and talents popping up every week as a result of being pushed by the work. Start now so you're confident later.

Writing your Descriptions

Our guidance from the personal statement section also applies here. However, when crafting your individual entries, each entry must include:

- *Title of your role*
- *Name of unit (i.e. team, lab, program)*
- *Institution name*
- *Date started and stopped*
- *Time commitment (in hours)*
- *Clear description of the activities undertaken by you*
- *Clear description of skills used, characteristics developed and qualities earned.*
- *Clear description of subjects (i.e. hospital patients, lower-year students, team members, etc.).*

AMCAS Work and Activities Summary

You should be consulting the AMCAS Instruction Manual for your application a year before preparing any element of your application but especially your sketch. The Work and Activities Sketch should include work experience, extracurricular activities, awards, honors, or publications.

You are permitted to make a total of 15 entries but you can enter four occurrences for each entry.

Of the 15 experiences, you can identify at least one but up to three that you consider to be your most meaningful experiences. By indicating that an entry is one of your most meaningful, the application will open up another 1325 characters that you can use to explain the nature of this experience. This is where the letter you received from your contact will be very useful. You can use it to describe what you did, why it mattered, what you learned and how you demonstrated the skills of a good doctor through the experience. Specifically, articulate the transformative nature of the experience both for you and the people you worked with.

Each activity must fit in one of these categories:

- *Paid employment (not military)*
- *Paid employment (military)*
- *Community service / volunteer (not medical / clinical)*
- *Community service / volunteer (medical / clinical)*
- *Research / lab*
- *Teaching / tutoring*
- *Honors / awards / recognitions*
- *Conferences attended*
- *Presentations / posters*
- *Publications*
- *Extracurricular / hobbies / avocations*
- *Leadership (not listed elsewhere)*
- *Intercollegiate athletics*
- *Artistic endeavors*
- *Other*

OMSAS Sketches

The Ontario medical schools that consider the sketch are the Northern Ontario School of Medicine, the University of Ottawa, Queen's University and the University of Toronto. McMaster and Western do not consider your sketch.

You can enter up to 48 items in your Autobiographical Sketch in seven categories: *employment, formal education, volunteer activities, extracurricular activities, awards and accomplishments, research and other.* Once you enter an item into the Sketch portal on OMSAS, you will be prompted to add details. Ideally, you've got a spreadsheet with the essential details already made up and it is just a matter of data entry and fact checking. You have 150 characters to describe each entry. Your goal should be to describe clearly the activity and your role. If there is space, you can add the attributes and qualities that you demonstrated through that entry.

The experiences can be both structured and non-structured, which is basically the distinction between formal and informal. You will need to assign a verifier to each activity listed. The verifiers can be added by clicking the View/Update Verifier button.

Selecting Verifiers

Entering the contact information for 48 reliable people can be an administrative disaster. This is why you should keep an up to date list of verifiers so that it is easy to access the information you need about the people who can attest to your activities.

Table: Sample Verifier Contact Information Tracker

Activity	Category	Entry #	Verifier Name	Title	Mailing Address	Email	Telephone Number

The ideal verifier is someone who held a leadership role in the activity listed, either as your boss, professor or superior. For Awards, the ideal verifier is the awards officer at the granting office. For sports or bands, the ideal verifier is a coach. For clinical experiences, the verifier should be the clinician themselves with their administrative assistant's phone number and email. If the experience took place 10 years ago, and you have lost touch with the verifier, it may be reasonable to leave this activity off of your sketch depending on how well it fits the criteria for best sketch entries above.

[SKETCH AND ESSAY SAMPLES CAN BE FOUND AT THE RESOURCE CHAPTER]

CASPer

This is a fairly new player on the scene of MD admissions in North America. McMaster University started testing CASPer in 2008/09 and implemented the 90-minute, web-based test for the first time in the 2010/11 application cycle. It has since become an independently run test and is becoming used more and more frequently by MD admissions committees across North America. The use and weight of CASPer for admissions varies. For further details about CASPer and preparing for your CASPer test, please refer to Chapter VI.

Interviews

We have an entire chapter dedicated to interviews and interview performance. This is a crucial step to gaining acceptance to medical school across North America. Interviews vary at every institution, though there are a few basic formats and key questions that every applicant must anticipate. Please see the chapter on Interview preparation for further details.

Letters of Recommendation/Reference Letters

Reference Letters or Letters of Evaluation aim to provide schools an insider's view of your professional capacities, your learning style and your ability to undertake medical training.

The best referees are:

- *Professors from upper year courses where you had a lot of one-on-one engagement.*

- *Physicians who have supervised you in clinical research or other activities*
- *Volunteer coordinators or managers who have worked with you over several years on a meaningful experience*
- *Principal investigators of labs in which you've spent at least 12 months, or graduate school supervisors.*
- *Employers in your most meaningful work experiences*
- *Coaches from meaningful team experiences*

AMCAS

For AMCAS, try to match your requested letters as closely as possible to the three most meaningful experiences on your sketch. These three experiences, along with three letters, will provide a crystal clear picture of who you may be as a doctor. This is, again, the entire goal of the medical school admissions process.

The referees from your three most meaningful experiences are likely the people who have seen you at your most passionate, your most engaged and your most skilled moments. If you feel that letters from these experiences aren't a good fit, then find another letter from someone who has witnessed the best of your attributes.

Review the AMCAS Instruction Manual carefully, ensuring you have the most current version, including the FAQs on letters, before requesting your letters.

OMSAS

OMSAS requires three Confidential Assessment Forms with letters from three Referees to go with your application. They should be submitted directly to OMSAS and not the schools themselves. There are clear and explicit instructions available through the OMSAS portal.

Asking Your Referees

You should request letters from referees at least eight weeks in advance of the deadline. If you have a commitment that is ending several months before your application, then ask first in person as the commitment is ending and then again via email at least eight weeks in advance of the deadline. Eight weeks is flexible enough to fit in around other deadlines, vacations, exams and teaching but not so long that the referees commit and then forget.

You can use these phrases to ask your referee in person to serve as a reference:

- *I would like you to be a referee for my application to medical school. Do you think you would be able to write me a strong, supportive letter?*
- *I am interested in discussing my application to medical school with you. I am wondering if you are interested in writing me a strong, supportive letter?*
- *I would be so grateful for a strong, supportive letter from you as part of my application to medical school. Is this something you feel confident doing?*

You can use this template (modify to use your own words) to ask your referee via email to serve as a reference:

Hello [Name],
I hope everything is well with [the lab, team, etc.].
I am writing to follow up from our discussion a few months ago around my application to medical school. I hope you're still able to write a strong, supportive letter to submit with my application.
I wanted you to know how meaningful our work was to my development as a [leader, learner, academic, etc.]. I benefited from [experience] in that I [list 1-2 items you learned or see differently now].
[Insert technical details, links and directions to submit letter]
I am happy to provide whatever support I can with this. I really appreciate it. Please let me know if the situation has changed and you are no longer able to write the letter.
Otherwise, I hope everything goes very well this [semester, season, etc.]. I will follow up in a few weeks to see how things are going.
Thanks again.

[Name]
[Email/ Phone #]

If you don't know if you are going to get a strong letter, try to select a different referee about whose recommendation you are more confident. However, there are some must-have referees. If you have completed a Master's or PhD, you must have a letter from your supervisor. An application without this letter raises huge red flags, even if you performed well in your degree. If you have been working in a lab for three years, you must have a letter from the principal investigator, or your team leader.

If you have a special consideration, a letter from someone who mentored or supported you through that difficult time that can attest to your fortitude, tenacity and grit is highly recommended. Ideally, this person is in a leadership role with some degree of repute so that the university can place the recommendation in context.

Special Consideration
Holistic admissions processes reflect the concept of "distance traveled" which is described by the AAMC as follows:

"Admissions officers are likely to place significance on any obstacles or hardships you've overcome to get to this point in your education. This is a concept known as "distance traveled" and medical schools view the challenges you've faced and conquered as admirable experience – and indicative of some very positive traits. As with other experiences, you can help the admissions committee better understand and appreciate your unique contributions by not only describing the experience, but also what you learned from this perspective."

Some schools do offer special consideration for people who have led more complex lives and have been required to take courses part-time or at several institutions. Not every school cares about distance traveled. This is why school selection must be done carefully with a strong filter.

If you are applying to a special program stream – such as those for Aboriginal applicants in Canada – then there will be additional requirements for submission of your application. We cannot review these for the 162 schools in North America but the opportunities for acceptance do exist if you're willing to explain your situation. For more on special consideration, see the Chapter on Non-Traditional and Mature Students.

CHAPTER IV

MCAT Overview

O ne of the most crucial components of a successful medical school application is a strong MCAT score. The Medical College Aptitude Test (MCAT) has been specifically designed to assess a candidate's "problem solving, critical thinking, and knowledge of natural, behavioral, and social science concepts and principles prerequisite to the study of medicine" (As per the AAMC, the administrating body for the MCAT). Essentially, through the MCAT and your performance on it, medical school admissions committees gain insight into your cognitive capacities, your didactic potential, and whether or not you have a solid foundational base to build upon once in medical school. By demonstrating your cognitive skills and your firm grasp of the fundamental sciences, and more importantly by scoring in the top ten percentile, you will assure medical schools that you will perform well in their rigorous academic programs.

In this chapter, we will share some important information that will help you plan effectively for your MCAT. We will also direct you to some very useful resources that can further assist you on your preparation journey. In the next chapter, we will go over a more in depth analysis of the Critical Analysis and Reasoning (CARS) section of the MCAT.

Know your enemy!

The first thing you should do is to intimately familiarize yourself with the American Association of Medical Colleges (AAMC) who is the official MCAT test provider. You can find them at the following URL: https://students-residents.aamc.org/applying-medical-school/taking-mcat-exam/

On their website, you will find ample information about the test. For example, you can find out when the test is available, how to register, etc. You can also read about the structure and format of the test: in fact, you can even get a minute-by-minute description of the test and how it is administered. More importantly, you will find valuable resources about what content will be covered on the test and how you should prepare for them. For instance, the *MCAT Essentials* section found on the AAMC website, which is updated annually, contains everything you need to know about the MCAT. You will find ample resources to help you prepare and there are lots of study materials for you to access such as sample question banks, link to organizations that provide MCAT study material, and more!

As indicated by the AAMC, "At the time of registration and on test day, you will be asked to certify that you have read, understand, and agree to comply with the policies and procedures contained within *The MCAT Essentials*." So before you do anything, make sure you visit the AAMC's website and read everything there is to read about the MCAT. This will help you plan your course of preparation much more efficiently as you will know exactly what to expect. The idea is to be able to reverse engineer your path so that by the time the MCAT comes around, you would have already done advance preparation, for example, by taking the appropriate courses that would have given you the knowledge base needed for the various sections of the test. This is the topic of the next section in this chapter.

The MCAT structure

To give you a general overview of the MCAT, it is divided into four sections that are discussed in more detail below. The entire exam is multiple choice with four answer choices (A, B, C, D) for each question. The questions are either based on a written passage or serve as stand-alone multiple-choice questions. You are allotted 95 minutes for each section (90 minutes for Critical Analysis and Reasoning Skills or CARS) with an optional 10-minute break between each section. The time allotted is section specific: you cannot carry over time or take time from one section for another (e.g. you are not permitted to finish the Biology section 10 minutes early to have 10 minutes more for CARS). All this material is covered in exhaustive detail in *The MCAT Essentials.*

The sections of the MCAT are detailed below:

1. **Chemical and Physical Foundations of Biological Systems**: This is the Chemistry/Physics section majorly though some questions will draw concepts from biology and organic chemistry as well. This section consists of 59 multiple-choice questions and you will have a total of 95 minutes to complete it. Note that, "most questions are organized around a descriptive passage. The other questions are not based on a descriptive passage and are independent of each other." All together there are 10 passage-based sets of questions (4-6 questions per set), and a total of 15 independent questions.

2. **Biological and Biochemical Foundations of Living systems**: This is the section where traditional "pre-med" applicants typically excel: no surprise there considering that this is the Biology section. The tricky thing with this section is that the MCAT test writers know that most traditional applicants will have covered this material in prior coursework and so take more liberty with varying the difficulty of the material. For example, some questions may be about glycolysis, a traditionally introductory level biochemistry concept whilst another questions may be about neurophysiology, a much more advanced topic. Don't worry about trying to cover every possible extensive detail here:, your goal will be to cover "enough" of the core material to obtain a good score. This 95-minute-long section also contains 59 questions in total, 10 of which are passage-based (4-6 questions per set), and 15 of which are independent questions.

3. **Critical Analysis and Reasoning Skills (CARS)**: This is arguably the most important section of the MCAT and is also the one that students typically struggle the most with. We have dedicated the entire next chapter to discuss this section in detail. Briefly, CARS contains a total of 53 questions designed around 9 passages that are to be answered in 90 minutes, requires you to read passages

from a variety of discourses such as the humanities, the social sciences, economics, politics, philosophy, etc.

4. **Psychological, Social, and Biological Foundations of Behavior**: This section was the newest addition to the MCAT when it was revamped in 2015. It tests concepts drawn from psychology, sociology, and other behavioral sciences. For example, you may be asked to answer a passage regarding the effects of poverty on rising rates of diabetes (thus showing an understanding of the social determinants of health) or be asked to identify the confirmation bias exhibited by a writer (a concept from social psychology). This section contains 59 questions. Fifteen of the questions will be independent while the remainder will be based around 10 passages. You will have a total 95 minutes to complete this section.

Preparing for the MCAT

As with any test or really, anything in life the key to success lies within preparation. Broadly speaking, preparation falls into two major categories: knowing the test and knowing the content. Knowing the test means becoming familiar with the actual exam itself: the test format, the structure of the test, and other areas regarding the actual administration and delivery of the test. This is achieved through reviewing materials such as The MCAT Essentials but comes more concretely from doing lots and lots of practice tests. The second part for preparation is in knowing the content. This latter part is where you will focus the majority of your time; this is what the "studying" part that most students think of with regard to the MCAT and what we will focus on.

It is definitely advantageous to have reviewed the materials covered on the MCAT in prior coursework. The good news here is that the majority of MCAT content is covered in introductory courses (i.e. mostly 1st and some 2nd year courses). These are your typical first year courses in introductory physics, organic chemistry, physical chemistry, biology, biochemistry, and psychology. Each institution offers a variation of these courses and it may be a good idea to consult your institutions course calendar and compare it to the concepts described in *The MCAT Essentials* to choose the best course for you.

While having taken these courses is a nice boost to your studying for the MCAT, having covered the material in prior coursework is by no means a requirement to succeed. Indeed, *The MCAT Essentials* offers a list of study resources for you to consult and study from whether or not you have encountered these concepts before.

When to take the MCAT?

This is a hotly debated topic and there is no clear answer other than the wonderfully useless advice that "the best time to write the MCAT is when you're ready!" There is a kernel of truth in this statement in that you should NOT write the MCAT unless you feel ready, don't try to push yourself to meet some fabricated deadline or feel that you must write the MCAT by x time. Write it when you're ready, are adequately prepared, and are positioned to succeed. That means you should write the test only when you are consistently scoring within your ideal score range during your practice tests. For a majority of traditional applicants, the summer after second year presents a great option. This is for two main reasons. First, by the summer of second year you will have covered a majority of the content through prior coursework. Second, doing the MCAT in the summer lets you dedicate more time and energy when you're not encumbered with trying to keep up with your other coursework and optimizing your GPA (which should always remain the priority).

Usually, preparing and taking the MCAT will occupy the majority of your time during the summer. It will almost feel like a full time job. So make sure that you do not have anything else planned that will occupy a large percentage of your time. This doesn't mean you put the rest of your life on hold, but you will need to realize that preparing for the MCAT will require a considerable amount of time, attention and resources. Whether you are enrolling in a prep-course or simply purchasing the study material and mock exams to prepare on your own, you will typically need to study 5-8 hours a day, 5 days a week for about 8-12 weeks in order to be fully prepared for the exam. Of course, this timeline will vary from individual to individual, but this timeframe is based on an average of several former candidates (now physicians) who have been very successful on their MCAT.

Once you have completed your preparations, at the end of the summer, you will write your MCAT. If things go well, great! If things do not go well, then you will have the opportunity to re-write the MCAT without losing an entire year as you will still be able to register for the late September sittings. A good way to gauge whether or not you're ready to write the MCAT is doing the mock-exams offered by the AAMC under real, life-like exam settings. If you do so and are scoring in the top 10th percentile consistently, you are likely ready.

The use of realistic mock exams under conditions that closely mimic actual test day conditions is of paramount importance. One of the biggest mistakes some students (specifically those who study on their own) make while preparing for the MCAT is to only practice sample questions in an unorganized manner without the restrictive conditions imposed by the actual test. You not only need to time yourself for each section, but you will need to develop the mental endurance to sit through an entire exam, from beginning to end. Therefore, you need to perform mock exams in their entirety so that you do not experience mental fatigue and burnout during the real exam. In fact you should go as far as doing your mock practice tests in a public place to mimic the distraction of having others around you, which will be unavoidable during your actual test.

Should I take a prep course?

We have superficially touched on this important question in the above sections and at this point it should not come as any surprise that we are entirely in favor of prep classes as a means to maximizing your performance on the MCAT.

So why do we find prep courses effective? Well, it all comes back to the notion and philosophy of functional training. Just like any other skill set, doing well on the MCAT (or CASPer, or your Multiple Mini Interview) requires some specific skills, and the best way to train those skill sets is by doing actual test that re-create the real test setting. In other words, your training must be functionally identical to the demands faced during actual test day conditions. Hence the benefit of prep programs, since they offer you the chance to practice using realistic mock MCAT simulations (N.B. this is aside from positive aspects of a structured learning environment, access to study material and instructors, access to question banks, etc.).

With that said, to use a prep company or to not use a prep company as part of your strategy for acing the MCAT depends entirely on you as an applicant. If you are the type of student who likes to have a structured learning environment and thrives under a rigorous schedule, then the prep course is for you. On the other hand, if you are an independent learner who finds success through self-directed learning strategies, then you can still be successful on the MCAT without enrolling in a prep course, but it will require some real discipline. Aside from that, all you will need is access to study material and question sets. And these are all readily available through any prep company or for free from such organizations as the Agha Khan Foundation. Whatever you do, do NOT skimp on preparation, again, if you have to invest, you have to invest and it is negligible compared to the cost of your education as a medical student.

The right attitude

Hopefully, having done all of the above, by the time your MCAT rolls around you are absolutely prepared and confident. A sense of confidence is the most important aspect of performing well in any setting and the MCAT is no different. Remind yourself that you have taken all of the appropriate courses, studied the relevant material, read widely outside of your scope, and spent ample time to prepare. Furthermore, recall that the MCAT is nothing more than a rudimentary examination of first year introductory material; concepts that you should have mastered inside and out by then.

Along the same line, the MCAT is a simple multiple-choice exam and when compared to other multiple-choice exams you may have seen (you know, the ones with 8 options) during your undergraduate years, it is much easier to approach. Lastly, if you are really dedicated to becoming a doctor, then you will surely realize that writing the MCAT will not be the most challenging thing you will have to do on your journey. So relax, take a deep breath, and realize this is just a simple test. You are already prepared!

In the next chapter we'll go into more preparation details about the most challenging part of the MCAT, the CARS section.

CHAPTER V

CARS, Drive to Success

With few exceptions, the Critical Analysis and Reasoning Skills (CARS) section is the single most frustrating section for most MCAT writers. Why? Well, it is arguably the only section that is truly skills-based rather than knowledge-based: the CARS section is testing your ability to perform a task rather than what you know or can apply. Before we offer a more in depth analysis of what CARS is testing, we better go over and stress the importance of the CARS section and why you should care.

Why CARS is the most important section

Simply put, CARS is the most important section of the MCAT. Why? **Because it's the one admissions committees use most frequently.** Several medical schools in North America currently only consider the CARS section of the MCAT. Several others deliberately set a much higher CARS cut off (scores in the 90th+ percentile), compared to other sections. This latter point is because of the way CARS is scored.

Look at the score table below adapted from the AAMC:

Score	Physical (Percentile Rank)	CARS (Percentile Rank)	Biological (Percentile Rank)	Psychological (Percentile Rank)
132	100	**100**	100	100

131	99	**99**	99	99
130	97	**98**	97	96
129	92	**95**	91	91
128	86	**90**	85	84
127	78	**83**	75	75
126	67	**72**	65	64
125	56	**61**	54	52

As you can see, the percentile rank required for a given score, is higher in CARS than the other sections. For example, if you scored in the 91-93rd percentile for all sections (a great job!), your score would be Physical 129, Biological 129, Psychological 129, and **CARS 128**. Your CARS score would be lower than the other sections even though you performed just as well; this is a function of the harsh score scaling used for CARS. Another way to look at this is the number of mistakes allowed per section to achieve a certain score. For a score of 129 in all the other sections, you are typically allowed 4-6 mistakes. **For a score of 129 in CARS, you are only permitted to get 3-4 wrong answers.** This varies by test and depends on the pre-determined scoring scale for your particular sitting. In general, to consistently and securely obtain a score above 128 (which is a great score and what you will be aiming for) you should aim to get no more than 4-5 answers wrong for the entire section.

General strategy

There are a ton of different strategies advocated by various prep companies centered on how to approach the CARS section. Be skeptical of everything you read about strategy/approaches (including this chapter!). The truth of the matter is that there is no one strategy that will work for everyone. Some people really flourish and do well with identifying different question types and structuring their practice around this. Others just start practicing and score 129 on their first ever mock MCAT CARS section (and yes, the authors of this chapter are just as envious as you of these "geniuses"). To sum it up, whatever strategy you use to tackle the MCAT CARS section needs to be tailored and modified to meet your needs.

This being said, there are some themes that emerge from success-ful candidates with regard to the MCAT CARS section. We will discuss a brief strategy for beginner, intermediate, and advanced applicants later in this chapter. Other than the general advice that you should read the entire passage without skimming and to read every question and answer choice carefully, we will discuss some more specific strategy items. The two main strategic tools that will benefit almost every candidate: under-standing the passage thesis and mastering the process of elimination.

The passage thesis

The passage thesis is the main idea, bottom line, main point, or what-ever else you want to call it of the passage: in essence, it's what the passage is about. The best way to think of this is as follows: it's a quick summary of the passage that captures the main points of the passage. For example, pretend you just read an article on the front page of the New York Times and ran into a friend in the elevator, how would you summarize this article to your friend within 10-15 seconds? What would it involve? Your summary is likely to include the 5 W's (who, what, where, when, why) as well as any other key information pertaining to the author and any potential biases they may have, if it was a balanced piece or very biased, etc. It's no surprise that this is an essential skill for CARS as by understanding the passage thesis means that in essence, you understand the entire passage. And after all, how could you possi-bly be asked to reason and think critically if you don't even understand the material?

You're probably thinking, "Alright, this doesn't sound so bad. I can read an article and summarize it. But these CARS passages aren't just like any normal article, they're...well, crazy hard!" And yes, you are com-pletely right. They are written this way on purpose. To be convoluted with terrible diction, innovative syntax, and often deploy a whole myriad of quirks related to the English language (much like this sentence!). Mastering the passage thesis is the most important and also the most time consuming skill you will need to develop. Remind yourself when you come across phrases or sections that just sound absurd, you are read-ing for general comprehension (to get the quick snapshot meaning of the passage), if you need to gloss over certain words or phrases, that's fine! Make a quick mental (and physical, if you wish) note that you didn't really understand this part but then move on with the rest of the passage.

The only way to get better at mastering the passage thesis (as with anything in life), is through practice. Practice doing as many CARS passages as you can get your hand on. Start reading material you otherwise wouldn't. A great way to practice is to start browsing through articles in high-level media sources such as The Economist, Philosophy Now, the New York Times, the Atlantic, the Globe and Mail, the Guardian (and whatever else your favorite/least favorite media source might be) and try to summarize these articles in your head after reading them. More on this in the next section.

Mastering the process of elimination

The process of elimination (POE) is going to be your best friend for the entire MCAT, especially for the CARS section. The POE for the CARS section is a multi-step process for most people. After you have read the passage (and I strongly advocate that you read the passage before you look at the question although this is a more flexible part of the strategy that you can tailor), go through the questions in order and eliminate the **obviously wrong** answer choices only. That means on your first pass of the question, you only eliminate answer choices that you for sure know to be wrong. Sometimes this allows you to eliminate 3 choices, thereby leaving you the correct answer (not likely and not often). Often, on your first pass you are only going to be able to eliminate 1 or maybe 2 choices. Your first pass should be very quick, remember, you are only looking for obviously wrong answers.

With the remaining answer choices, your job is to find the most correct answer. Don't you hate that? The "most correct" or "least wrong." But that's the entire point of the CARS section, to test how you handle uncertainty and reason when there is no concrete answer available (as we physicians do 90% of the time). With the remainder of your answer choices (often all 4), you undergo what I like to call the second pass. In this second pass, you are carefully examining the answer choices for logical fallacies, incongruences with the author's views, and most importantly, inconsistencies with the passage thesis. This is when you compare each answer choice to the question (make sure it answers the question and isn't just a nonsensical answer), the passage thesis, and other answer choices (if for example answers A and B are exact opposites of each other, then it is likely that one of them is correct given that they answer the question appropriately).

It's very hard to describe the art involved in the process of elimination in a book format that's going to be effective for every student. Some of the most common mistakes include eliminating answer choices that aren't obviously wrong on the first pass, not understanding/carefully reading the question and answer choices, as well as logical fallacies (e.g. not correctly identifying which answer choice is a bigger leap of inference versus another answer choice).

Beginner, Intermediate, and Advanced Strategies
As you can tell, the advice given in this section is very general. That is necessary for a book such as this because it is meant to target a range of audience including those who have never taken a practice CARS test before to those who are seasoned veterans scoring between 126-128, trying to bust through that ceiling (more on that later). There are certain patterns of thinking and common pitfalls that candidates fall in depending on where they are scoring. We have tried to summarize these below for you. Keep in mind that these are still generalities and no amount of generalized written information can substitute a personalized study/strategy plan tailored for you:

Beginner (Score 118-122)

- *Missing entire passages and/or large portions of passages*
- *Focus should be on reading comprehension and developing a good understanding of the passage thesis*
- *Practice reading and summarizing more social science and humanities literature, especially topics that are unfamiliar. Some good sources including the Economist, Philosophy Now, or other high-level media sources*
- *Begin practicing the process of elimination but main focus should remain on understanding the passage thesis*

- *Understanding the passage thesis.* Have we emphasized this enough yet? *Practice, practice, practice.*

Intermediate (Score 123-127)

- *Generally fall into one of two categories: missing most of a single passage or missing a few questions across all passages*
- *If missing most of a single passage, focus should remain on understanding the passage thesis. Practice by reading more challenging items from sources such as The Economist or Philosophy Now.*
- *If missing few questions across all passages, carefully go over every single question from practice passages (even the ones you got right). Make sure you understand why every answer choice that is incorrect is wrong and why the correct one makes sense. If you don't understand certain items, talk through it with an expert.*
- *For questions that you got wrong, don't look at the answer guide. See if you can logic out what the right answer is, how you came to your answer, and why your method was incorrect.*
- *See the section below about busting through the "128 ceiling"*

Advanced (Score 128+)

- *Consistency is key here, continue to practice and carefully go over every single question in a practice exam*
- *At this level, the kind of mistakes that people make are very specific and individualized, consider consulting an expert for specific and tailored feedback*

How to practice

Depending on which category (beginner, intermediate, or advanced) you fall into, the way you practice is going to vary. Generally speaking, if you are a beginner, the focus should be on reading comprehension, on really getting the passage thesis down. When practicing with individual passages at this stage, don't worry about trying to maintain a time limit.

Do time yourself just so you know how much you are spending per passage. That being said, **always do entire practice exams adhering to the actual time limit**. You are given 90 minutes for the CARS section with 9 passages (averaging to about 10 minutes a passage). We recommend doing a full practice exam once a week at this stage.

For those of you falling into the intermediate level, the bulk of your practice should be centered on entire practice exams under timed circumstances. The CARS section is very time constrained. You should be practicing in as close to real-life circumstances as possible at this point (i.e. taking these tests in a quiet but not silent setting). The pace suitable for most people is about 2 full practice exams per week. The majority of your time will be spent going over these exams in detail through the week, reviewing every single question and understanding why an answer choice is correct or incorrect.

Be careful not to fall into the trap of only reviewing questions you got wrong or thinking "oh that's a silly mistake that I won't make on my real MCAT." If you made the mistake in practice, chances are you're going to make it on the real thing. That's why it's important to treat each of these practice exams as if it's the real deal. Be diligent in reviewing these practice exams, it should be taking you at least twice to three times as long to review each exam as the time spent actually doing it.

Busting through the "128 ceiling"

You will notice that many MCAT prep companies and articles you read about the CARS section will focus on the beginner/intermediate score range. This is because to achieve scores above 128, it is very difficult to offer general advice and tips that will work for everybody. For the advanced range scores above 128, the practice is all going to be about consistency and detail. That means being extra thorough when reviewing practice exams and fully understanding each and every question/answer choice. For every mistake made on practice, you need to be able to fully understand why it was you made this mistake, the thinking that got you there, and the logic trap you fell for. There is no cookie-cutter solution at this level of the game; you really need expert advice and feedback. Something that would definitely help at this stage is reading a book on logical fallacies and becoming familiar with identifying different types of fallacies and how to avoid them.

Example MCAT CARS Passage

We're now ready to tackle a sample passage followed by detailed answers to each of the questions. (To get even more practice passages, visit https://bemoacademicconsulting.com/sample-mcat-cars to gain free access to 10 sample difficult passages and questions plus expert analysis and response.)

Sample passage:

Heralded as the father of existentialism, Kierkegaard's debut work of influence *Either/Or* presents the categorical existence of two spheres, the aesthetic and the ethical. The hedonistic, distractible stage of aesthetic living is governed by circumstances of moment, where one fleeting event – such as the smile of a pretty girl – leads to the next and so too does the motif for the aesthetic's fantasy. The ethical sphere is entered when the nature and judgments of one's choices are considered. Individual agency, whilst present before, truly manifests in bearing the responsibility of one's good or bad choices.

For Kierkegaard, the ethical sphere was intimately connected with the religious sphere explored in his subsequent works. Whilst the ethical has a commitment with morality, the religious is a covenant with God. It is based on faith; Christianity is seen as truth, although Kierkegaard admits it to be paradoxical and oppositional to logic. It is through conscious choice that movement from the ethical sphere to the religious occurs – with a leap of faith. Despite a seeming progression implied in Kierkegaard's works, the spheres are not independent entities exclusive of each other. One who lives primarily in the religious sphere, for example, will still have aspects of her being enjoying fleeting moments of beauty and have morality govern her choices.

Kierkegaard's leap of faith is denounced by his successor, Sartre, who rejects the notion of divine orchestration, tarring such leaps as bad faith. Moreover, Sartre vehemently argues for the oppressive nature of social constructs and collectivist forces that usher the individual into rejecting his or her innate freedom for that of the greater good. It is this narrowing and limiting of choice that Sartre defined as bad faith. In a manner, any and all external influences that cause one to live in an inauthentic fashion – such as the social scripts followed on a first date, in a restaurant – are judged to be guilty and worthy of re-examination.

The core of Sartre's philosophies hinge upon the oft quoted adage, "existence proceeds essence." It is man who first and foremost is before he defines the parameters of that existence through conscious and deliberate choice. It is therefore of no consequence the station, nature, and parameters surrounding one's birth when considering the nature of one's being. Essence is defined through choice. But how can one make such a choice when the options are seemingly limitless and each has unbeknownst consequences? Indeed, it is so daunting an experience that Sartre dubbed this Existential Angst.

In an elegant application of existential philosophy, a former concentration camp prisoner, Frankl, posits that regardless of how harsh, cruel, and inhumane the external environment may be, one's inner state and reaction is defined by agency. He defines this internal state and motivation as one's attitude in relation to outside circumstance. Of paramount importance for Frankl is finding and making meaning of the circumstances in one's life. The application of his philosophy in action is what gives Frankl's narrative its power. Where Kierkegaard and Sartre's philosophies were also deeply personal and practical, they were nonetheless born out of academia. Frankl's insightful analysis and presentation of the prisoner's internal state was a lived experience, lending it to be more accessible for the layperson.

Sample MCAT CARS Questions

1. What is Existential Angst (paragraph 4)?

a. The feelings one has when confronted with choice
b. The state of desperation when contemplating that existence proceeds essence

c. The task of making seemingly limitless choices

d. The anxiety and regret associated with having made a choice

2. The author would most agree with which of the following statements:

a. Existentialism is a philosophy about agency and choice, best introduced through reading passages such as this one

b. Frankl's philosophy is better than Kierkegaard and Sartre's

c. Kierkegaard and Sartre's philosophies were impractical when compared to Frankl's philosophy

d. Applying the principles of existentialism to everyday life is better than just talking about it

3. Which of the following best describes the main goal of the passage?

a. To compare the different philosophies of Kierkegaard, Sartre, and Frankl

b. To show a progression of existential philosophy

c. To demonstrate how existentialism has changed with time

d. To offer an introduction to existential philosophy

4. According to the passage's depiction of Kierkegaard, which of the following policies would he most support?

a. That students should have the choice to attend either a secular or religious school

b. That Existentialism should be taught in schools

c. That World Religions should be taught in schools

d. That public funding should be provided for religious school boards

5. Which of the following statements is least supported by the passage?

a. Sartre believed men and women were equals
b. Sartre supported laws to prevent discrimination
c. Sartre believed that a poor man could become rich if he worked hard enough
d. Sartre was denounced by the church

Answers

1. What is Existential Angst (paragraph 4)?

a. The feelings one has when confronted with choice
b. The state of desperation when contemplating that existence proceeds essence
c. The task of making seemingly limitless choices
d. The anxiety and regret associated with having made a choice

This is a comprehension question. It is best approached through going to the text and having a clear understanding and definition for the term in question. Existential Angst is described in the passage as the "daunting experience" of making a choice when "options are seemingly limitless." Important here are two things:

1. That it is an experience (i.e. a state, an emotion, a feeling) and
2. That it is the emotion felt when having to make a choice (i.e. the process of choosing).

A: This is correct as it has both parts: the experience (feelings) felt when confronted (having to make) a choice
B: The first part of this answer is correct, as a state of desperation is definitely a feeling. However, the second part of this answer is not

relevant, as Sartre never linked Existential Angst to his adage that was "existence proceeds essence"

C: The first part of this answer is incorrect as Existential Angst is about the experience when confronted with choice, not the task of making choices

D: This answer stem is incorrect as it is in the past tense. It relates the anxiety and regret (both which would be legitimate feelings for Existential Angst) to choices that have already been made, not choices that are currently available.

2. The author would most agree with which of the following statements:

a. Existentialism is a philosophy about agency and choice, best introduced through reading passages such as this one

b. Frankl's philosophy is better than Kierkegaard and Sartre's

c. Kierkegaard and Sartre's philosophies were impractical when compared to Frankl's philosophy

d. Applying the principles of existentialism to everyday life is better than just talking about it

This is a "Reasoning Beyond the Text" question. It is best approached through process of elimination. Note that the tone of the last paragraph is immensely positive when compared the rather neutral tone for the rest of the passage. Also, although this last paragraph seems to focus on Frankl's philosophy, upon further scrutiny the positivity associated with the paragraph is actually for the APPLICATION of Frankl's philosophy. This question is best approached using your understanding of the thesis (main goal) of the passage and process of elimination.

A: The first part of this answer characterizing Existentialism is correct. However, the author states that part of Frankl's philosophies effectiveness is that it is a "lived experience" and more accessible this way. This implies that Existentialism is best taught through real life experiences rather than reading.

B: Although it may seem that the author is stating that Frankl's philosophies are better with the positive tone in the last paragraph, it is rather the APPLICATION of Frankl's philosophies that the author is praising, not his philosophies itself.

C: This is an attractive answer choice, as the author seems to imply that because Kierkegaard and Sartre's philosophies were born out of academia, they're therefore less practical. However, the author does not actually compare the practicality of each of the respective philosophies, instead saying that Frankl's philosophy is merely more accessible (i.e. easier to understand) as it is presented as a lived experience rather than in academia, presumably as a textbook or lecture. The author does not comment on the practicality of Frankl's philosophy itself.

D: The entirety of the last paragraph is lavish with praise regarding the application of existential philosophy in Frankl's case. It is implied therefore that the author has a highly positive view of applications of existential philosophy.

3. Which of the following best describes the main goal of the passage?

a. To compare the different philosophies of Kierkegaard, Sartre, and Frankl

b. To show a progression of existential philosophy

c. To demonstrate how existentialism has changed with time

d. To offer an introduction to existential philosophy

This is a comprehension question directly asking for the main goal of the passage (i.e. what is this passage about?) This is best answered using your formulation of the thesis (main goal) of the passage and using process of elimination.

A: Although the author certainly discusses the philosophies of Kierkegaard, Sartre, and Frankl, he does not compare (i.e. drawing relationships between them, showing pros/cons, analyzing, etc.) them. Rather, the author just offers a brief overview of each of their philosophy.

B: There is a direct progression from Kierkegaard to Sartre (Kierkegaard's "successor" Paragraph 3) and an implied one in the last paragraph with Frankl as the author introduces Frankl as having applied existentialist principles, presumably introduced by Kierkegaard and Sartre.

C: Although the passage illustrates how various separate existentialist philosophies have developed, it does not make explicit a time component. Furthermore, the passage does not presume to offer a full overview of existentialism but rather traces a distinct progression for a few philosophers (choice B).

D: Again, the passage is not offering an overview of Existentialism as a whole as would be expected in an introduction. It focuses on three distinct philosophers and traces the author's take on a progression of existential thought.

4. According to the passage's depiction of Kierkegaard, which of the following policies would he most support?

a. That students should have the choice to attend either a secular or religious school
b. That Existentialism should be taught in schools
c. That World Religions should be taught in schools
d. That public funding should be provided for religious school boards

This is a "Reasoning Beyond the Text" question. The passages description of Kierkegaard is that he is concerned with individual agency and choice but only insofar as one's relation to God. It is directly stated, "Christianity is seen as truth" (paragraph 2). This question is best approached using process of elimination.

A: The author's depiction of Kierkegaard does emphasize agency and choice (the students choice), he nevertheless saw Christianity as truth. There is also an implicit progression or growth noted from the aesthetic, to the ethical, and ultimately the religious sphere. Therefore, Kierkegaard would most have supported that all students attend Christian (or religious) school where they would've become familiar with this truth.

B: According to the passage, Kierkegaard did not state that existentialism should be taught or even spread. Rather, it is merely an explanation and analysis for the way people are and might live.

C: Although Kierkegaard would certainly have supported teaching Christianity in schools, he would not have supported the teaching of World Religions or any other religions.

D: By providing funding for religious schools, they would be more accessible to more people. This includes Christian school boards that Kierkegaard would have supported for all students to attend, as he believed Christianity was truth.

5. Which of the following statements is least supported by the passage?

a. Sartre believed men and women were equals

b. Sartre supported laws to prevent discrimination

c. Sartre believed that a poor man could become rich if he worked hard enough

d. Sartre was denounced by the Church

This is a "Reasoning Beyond the Text" question. The passage describes Sartre as an a atheistic philosopher who was primarily concerned above all else with choice and freedom of choice: "It is this narrowing and limiting of choice that Sartre defined as bad faith... any and all external influences that cause one to live in an inauthentic fashion... are judged to be guilty" (paragraph 3). Be careful here as this question asks for the LEAST supported (i.e. the choice that has the biggest leap in logic or lowest amount of evidence). The process of elimination here works well.

A: This is supported by the passage as Sartre is said to believe that it is "of no consequence the station, nature, and parameters surrounding one's birth" (paragraph 4). This would imply that anything surrounding one's birth (such as one's sex) is not important and therefore equal.

B: Although Sartre may have believed that the nature of birth is of no consequence; he nevertheless strongly disagreed with social constructs and anything that limits choice (such as this law would).

C: This is a direct application of Sartre's philosophy as he believed that one's choices (such as hard work) were more important than the situation one was born into.

D: This can be inferred from the strong denunciation of faith and religion that Sartre expressed as "bad faith." It is logical to assume that the Church would have been in disagreement with Sartre.

CHAPTER VI

CASPer: McMaster's Best Kept "Secret!"

What is CASPer?

The Computer-based Assessment for Sampling Personal Characteristics (**CASPer**) is an online-based situational judgment test designed to assess how you approach and consider different real-life scenarios and the problems within them. The test was originally designed by McMaster University for screening their medical school applicants. Since then CASPer has been licensed to a for-profit corporation to administer the test, while McMaster University remains a part shareholder of this corporation. The test is currently used as part of the admissions process by several academic programs and is expected to be adopted by a limited number of programs until it is replaced by a more reliable test in the near future.

Unlike more traditional examinations, each scenario in CASPer is either described in a stanza of text, or in the form of a video clip. The candidate is then presented with three questions pertaining to each scenario. These questions are designed to assess how the candidate has considered the scenario and their approach to the unique challenges presented in each question. Importantly, the applicants only have a total of 5 minutes to answer all three questions for each scenario. The entire test consists of 12 such scenarios lasting 90 minutes in total.

Why devote an entire chapter to CASPer?

CASPer is unique and distinct from other methods of assessing personal characteristics such as traditional/panel interviews, personal statements, or references, in that it is claimed to provide assessors a tool free from subjective bias that can be used as an objective measure of professionalism.

CASPer claims to assess your ability to think quickly, critically, and fairly. The time constraints for responses on CASPer are designed to only allow snap decisions and quick judgments – you are only given 5 minutes by design. This way, the test hopes to assess your true, authentic reaction and decision making abilities without giving you the chance to give a well thought-out and crafted answer that may not actually reflect your real life behavior.

For the sake of completeness, it is important to note here that, in our opinion, although there has been some research pointing to the efficacy of CASPer as an admissions tool, the majority of such research has been done by the same researchers/university that have now turned the test into a for-profit company and, in our opinion, such claims must be viewed with caution until further independent studies have been conducted to verify CASPer's validity and/or efficacy.

Importantly, unlike CASPer creators' claims that the test might be "immune to coaching", we have cogent evidence that candidates who adequately and appropriately prepare and practice for this assessment are far more likely to score higher than those who do not. These are based on the results of BeMo's CASPer prep programs and our own independent research.

How to Prepare

1. Familiarize yourself with the test format

Sun Tzu, a Chinese military general once said "Every battle is won before it's ever fought". Knowing what you're up against before you encounter it has long been known to be a strategic advantage, and CASPer is no different.

What to expect:

a. 12 scenarios presented in the form of either a short written stem or a video clip, which is usually 2 minutes or less in length
b. 3 questions based around the stem in Short-Answer Question format
c. A total of 5 minutes to answer all 3 questions based on the scenario.

Your task is to provide answers to each of the questions that are based around the scenario by typing your responses into the text boxes of each question.

2. Understand what you need to demonstrate

The purpose of the test is to assess your interpersonal skills by presenting you with scenarios that challenge different aspects of your personality and character, and observing how you respond to these challenges. Your responses will be analyzed in how they demonstrate favorable characteristics (i.e. reflective appraisal, empathy, professionalism, ethical consideration, altruism) for medical school admission and to what extent they demonstrate this.

Whilst possessing these characteristics is a prerequisite for demonstrating them, we are assuming for the purposes of this text that you already possess them (in other words, we are not advocating for nor are we teaching you how to "fake it"). Demonstrating them is not always easy, and in the context of CASPer, requires practice. Each of these characteristics is demonstrable through answers to questions based on the scenarios you will encounter during your test. Whilst you don't need to demonstrate them all in every answer, certain situations will lend themselves to one or more than the others – learning how to recognize this and respond accordingly takes practice and expert guidance so that you can identify your weaknesses and learn from them.

Some questions will be posed so as to put you as the focus of the scenario and ask how you would respond when faced with this situation. Others will simply ask you to comment on your opinions of the scenario as a 3rd person observer. This shouldn't change your answer significantly, other than the phrasing of your answer (e.g. using "I would" rather than "he/she would", etc.). The important thing is to grasp what key issue is at play in the scenario and address it accordingly.

A great way to demonstrate you have a keen grasp of the underlying social or ethical issues of the scenarios presented is to provide a balanced (albeit brief) discussion of both sides of the argument, or both choices in a dichotomous decision (e.g. taking vs. not taking performance enhancing drugs). You don't need to write an essay on the topic, in fact this is usually limited by either the character count of the text boxes (which keeps changing or disappearing from year to year) or the time limit imposed on the questions. This demonstrates to your assessor that you are able to apply critical thinking to all aspects of a situation, even when there appears to be a clear-cut right and wrong answer – this is an important skill. If you respond overwhelmingly in favor of one course of action, this demonstrates conviction and confidence. This is best done however after offering a balanced investigation and deliberation of multiple sides of an issues.

Above all else, DO NOT profess support for a decision or course of action that will cause harm, be illegal, create conflict or be in any way unethical or unprofessional. The scenarios in the test you will be faced with may be completely unrelated to medicine, but the characteristics the test is analyzing are being used to determine your suitability to work in the medical profession. Any of the above contained within an answer is an instant red flag for your assessor and will leave you scoring low, if at all, on that question. In fact, the assessors are instructed to report such red flags.

3. Familiarize yourself with the types of scenarios you will face

CASPer is designed to assess your ability to make moral and ethical decisions in the face of a challenging set of circumstances or dilemmas. However, knowing this does not adequately prepare you to respond to the questions well. There are numerous possible scenarios you will be faced with, and each one will have nuances and details specific to that situation that must be considered and factored into your responses.

BeMo Academic Consulting has identified 16 distinct major types of question that you may be faced with during the CASPer test. They are as follows:

1. *Conflict of Interest*
2. *Ethical Dilemma*
3. *Professional Boundaries*
4. *Scope of Practice*
5. *Social/ Current Events Awareness*
6. *Personal Questions*
7. *Patient Autonomy*
8. *Evidence-based Practice*
9. *Informed Consent*
10. *Rural vs. City Practice*
11. *Medical Legal*
12. *Alternative Medicine*
13. *Non-judgmental Approach*
14. *Conflict Resolution*
15. *Global Health*
16. *Problem-based learning*

Although your approach to each scenario will be tailored specifically for that question, it is generally advisable to develop a framework for approaching each situation that will cover the important general aspects of the situation at hand. There is no one set framework that has been proven to be better than any other, and it is perfectly acceptable to develop your own guidelines that work effectively. However, most frameworks should include some consideration to each of the following:

- *What is the setting of the scenario and how will this affect my decision-making?*
- *What information is missing or is incomplete? (If gathering facts involves having a sensitive conversation with another individual, make sure you explicitly say that you will have a private conversation to ask questions in a non-judgmental manner.)*
- *Remain non-judgmental and do not make any hasty conclusions based on the primary evidence provided in the scenario.*
- *Who is directly or indirectly involved in the scenario and how will this affect my approach to each person?*
- *What are the unassailable facts of the case?*

- *How much of what has happened is opinion or conjecture?*
- *What is the key issue at play?*
- *What are the options available to me?*

4. Familiarize yourself with the medical ethics landscape

It is important to realize the context in which you are being assessed. Your responses to the questions in each scenario are being judged based on the ethical principles your assessors have learned and apply almost every day in their professional lives. It stands to reason then that, if you are familiar with these principles, you are ahead of the curve in this exam.

All prospective medical students should be well-read in general medical ethics principles in the jurisdiction that they will be writing the test. Aside from the myriad of ethics texts available, online resources such as any of the provincial or state licensing authority websites, American (or Canadian) Medical Protection Association (the medico-legal defense body for physicians in the US and Canada), the AAMC core competencies, the CanMEDS principles and MedlinePlus all have ample reading material relating to the ethical principles that apply to all physicians practicing in the United States, Canada and globally.

5. Practice with realistic CASPer simulations & get expert feedback

Situational judgment tests such as CASPer test behavioral skills; so just reading an ethics textbook is not sufficient preparation. Just like riding a bike or swimming, practice performing the task is essential to develop proficiency in it. You must repeatedly immerse yourself in moral and ethical dilemmas and challenge your own decision making within them. There are numerous resources available to facilitate this practice – many more modern ethics textbooks contain questions of a similar format to CASPer questions with discussions around the answers. BeMo Academic Consulting offers numerous resources in preparation for CASPer including a CASPer prep video course, realistic CASPer simulations (BeMo's CASPer SIM™ Tests) and opportunities for one-to-one expert feedback. (Visit BeMoAcademicConsulting.com to learn more).

The old adage, "practice makes perfect" is, in reality, somewhat misleading. Over the years, research has revealed that practice only makes permanent. The expression should really be "*perfect* practice makes perfect." If you perform a task incorrectly repeatedly, you will not become more proficient in it, rather your inappropriate behavior will simply turn into a bad habit. It is for this important reason that you need expert feedback as part of your learning cycle in order to improve. Feedback in this context should ideally come from someone highly experienced in considering ethical dilemmas, (a service we offer our students in our paid training programs - see above), however it would also be beneficial to organize group study sessions to discuss different ethical issues and how to approach them. This offers group feedback which, although not expert feedback, can help you identify ethical issues that some of the group individuals may not fully grasp.

Sample CASPer Scenarios

Although not an extensive list of questions, the ones presented below will allow you to practice some of the concepts you have learned, and will further learn, in this chapter. Have fun! Please note, that although the questions here are performed in written, text format, the majority of actual CASPer scenarios will be videos that demonstrate these concepts in one way or another. (To watch sample videos visit our CASPer resource site at https://caspertestprep.com/)

1) Countries that offer a 'one-payer' governmental healthcare system, one in which the access to healthcare and its services are free and open to all individuals without a costs, at times face economic pressures due to aging populations, excessive and inappropriate use of services such as visits to the ER for minor health issues, etc. As a means to combat and offset some of these growing financial costs, some countries have discussed introducing a $10 fee to be paid by the patients when they seek out medical care. What are your views about such a proposal and policy?

What are the implications of introducing a $10 fee, payable by patients?

2) You are shopping at the local grocery store. As you are going about your shopping, you notice an elderly lady in the same aisle taking items off the shelf and stuff them into her winter coat. Then, a store employee who had seen the same thing approaches the elderly lady and begins to accuse her of stealing. The store employee even points at you and says that you saw her do it as well and you are a witness. The lady seems very confused and does not know how to react. What would you do as the store manager in this situation if you were informed of what had transpired?

3) You are a truck driver waiting at the local bar where other drivers are hanging out, awaiting your next route. Knowing you are on duty you simply order a coffee and pie. You sit down next to another colleague, Jim, who tells you he is also awaiting his next route. In front of him you see several empty pints that have some left over beer. Your colleague gets a call informing him of his next assignment. You over hear him accept the assignment. What will you do in this situation?

4) You are a female professor. A male student of yours has been making more frequent visits to your office. You also sense that he is sharing too much of his personal life with you (talking about recent break-up) and being excessively friendly. He now brings you a coffee on each visit and asks you about your weekend plans. How should you deal with this student?

Top Tips for Acing the Test

Now that you have all the tools you need to be able to prepare for the test ahead of time, there are a number of strategies you need to have in the back of your mind when taking the test itself. The strategies will help you navigate the actual test more efficiently. More importantly, having strategies ahead of time allows you to feel less anxious while taking the test. Here are some tips:

1. Read each question twice before you provide your response to any question

Despite your time limit on each question, you are not so time pressured that you can't go over the questions again. Your goal is to first completely understand the question and decide which of the three questions is easier to tackle first, rather than responding in the same order they are presented. In most exams, candidates' nerves settle down after a few questions, but many are at risk of misreading or missing something from the first few questions and they do this purely because they are so nervous. Moreover, misunderstanding something crucial can be the difference between a stellar answer and a dreadful one which, in turn, can mean the difference between an average mark and a great one. Ensuring you have understood everything presented in the question pays huge dividends that you don't necessarily appreciate until you've fallen foul of this trap – avoid learning this lesson the hard way by taking the extra 30 seconds to fully absorb everything given to you.

2. Take time to consider your answer

In a similar way to re-reading the questions, taking a few moments to compose your thoughts and running through in your head how you want to word your response is a far better approach than typing down thoughts as they pop into your head. Although you won't be penalized for having a disorganized answer (provided it contains well-reasoned points), it will make the answer more difficult to read for the assessor that then prevents them from giving you top marks. Don't just start typing the second you've finished reading the questions, take a (brief) moment to get your head around what's going on and then begin responding.

3. Pay attention to your spelling and grammar

CASPer assessors are specifically told NOT to penalize candidates for spelling and grammar errors. This rule was designed to ensure that candidates are not penalized due to the time limit. Whilst that rule is adhered to within the scope of its intention, it is something of an impossibility for there not to be score discrepancies between answers with no spelling or grammar errors and those that do.

It is much easier than you may think to identify those whom English is not their first language (or generally have poor written communications skills in English), and those who speak fluent English based on CASPer answers. Whilst significant allowances are made for answers with misspelled words or inappropriately constructed sentences, it is far less likely that you will get your point across adequately to the assessor with an answer that contains either of these. That being said, a slip of the hand when typing an answer leading to two letters switching place in a word will not negatively impact your score.

4. Read your answers over again when you are finished (if time permits)

Not only does this help with the last point by picking up spelling mistakes you may not have noticed when you were typing your answers to the questions, but it allows you to double check that you are happy with what you wrote, how it reads and how it is presented. Although you may not have time to "draft" answers to all the questions to then go back and finalize each answer, you should definitely be able to re-read every answer before moving forward. Again, if time permits.

5. If you get stuck, stick to your framework

The general framework we talked about earlier that you should be able to apply to each scenario irrespective of its content should be burned into your brain by this point with all the practice you did! If you're faced with a scenario that you're unfamiliar with and are struggling to grasp, stop. Take a deep breath. Re-consider the question stem if necessary. Go back to your basics from your framework. Tackle each question one at a time.

Don't forget, if you finish a question and feel like you did poorly on it or you ran out of time, clear your head and move on. One or two bad scenarios with the rest going well still gives you a great chance of scoring high. Remember, each scenario is a new set of points to score, so you can definitely make up for low-scoring ones here and there.

6. It's OK if you completely miss a question or two in a given scenario

We won't expand upon this point at this juncture as the point will become very clear once you have read the subsequent section on how the test is scored.

How CASPer is marked

Possibly the most frequently asked question about CASPer is, "How is it scored?". While this isn't a secret *per se*, it is not something medical schools will actively provide you with, although the publicly available research by CASPer creators provides many hints. Keep in mind that knowing how the scoring system works is not the same (and not even as important) as knowing what the assessors are looking for when scoring the questions. It also shouldn't change your approach to the questions or how you construct your responses.

Each CASPer assessor is given an online orientation and training session on the logistical aspects of marking the tests (e.g. how to use the secure login system, how to ensure they have the appropriate software for running the media clips, etc.) and the criteria they must apply to each response when grading it. This is the aspect of the test that is claimed to minimize subjective judgment in favor of objective assessment criteria (notice that we use the term "minimize", not "remove"). Tests with written answers marked by humans, even ones who are experts in this field, will never be 100% objective, CASPer's use of old technology is not an exception, in our opinion.

The assessors for the test are individuals from all walks of life. They include medical professionals, medical students and residents, members of the public, undergraduate students, or anyone provided with a registration code which allows them go through the online training process and become a CASPer assessor.

The online training program gives an overview of the test and how it should be scored. Recall that, each assessor only sees one scenario for each applicant and they are not aware of the applicant's personal identifiers. Thus, each applicant's CASPer results will be seen by 12 distinct assessors, helping to increase the inter-observer reliability of the test. The assessors are given general information about the concepts important to each scenario and major ideas that should be discussed, but they are not provided with an answer key.

As the assessors analyze your responses, they will be applying the CASPer marking criteria to each answer. Application of the criteria will vary from question to question as, you may be given a scenario centered around informed consent, but then be asked a question on patient autonomy. Here is an example:

> Question 1: "You are a surgical resident in an outpatient clinic seeing a patient who has been diagnosed with ovarian cancer that requires surgical intervention. You are discussing the details of the surgery, and explain that both open and laparoscopic oophorectomy are possibilities in her case. How would you ensure any consent this patient provides for surgery is informed?"
>
> Follow-up Question: "After your discussion, the patient expresses that she does not wish to undergo surgery, stating that she would like to give chemotherapy a chance first. How would you respond to this decision?"

First note that advance technical knowledge of "open and laparoscopic oophorectomy" is irrelevant and if you see a technical term in CASPer it is just meant to shake you up a bit and stress you. As you can see, this sample question encompasses numerous areas and deals with several ethical concepts. While the first question specifically asks about informed consent, the second then adds a dimension of patient autonomy and could even be argued to branch into Evidence-based Medicine.

From an assessors' point of view, the more dimensions of the question you can demonstrate to have recognized and considered, the better the grade you will receive. In this example, you would need to appreciate what important aspects of the patient encounter contribute to informed consent (e.g. proposed procedure, details, possible alternatives, risks and complications, consequences of doing nothing, etc.) and recognizing that, provided the patient has the capacity to make their own decisions about their healthcare, that making the decision to decline surgery, although potentially inadvisable within the context of their illness, is a patient's inalienable right as part of their autonomy.

The grading of CASPer responses is done using a numerical Likert-style scale. The scale runs from 1 to 9 with 1 signifying a "unsatisfactory" response and 9 signifying a "superb" or superior one. Although all of your three responses to the questions for the same scenario will be graded by the same assessor, the score that you receive is representative of your overall performance on that station. For instance, if during one of the scenarios you take a lot of time to provide a well-thought out and mature answer to only one of the three questions and only have limited time (or no time at all) to answer the remaining two, you can still score high on that station, granted that the answer you provided to question one was strong, appropriate and professional.

Assessors are not required to comment on the score they give or provide any feedback justifying the score. However, they do have an option to flag a particular answer and/or indicate the possibility of technical glitches that may have led to a poor performance at a given station. (N.B: The CASPer system is claimed to be designed to detect technical problems and report it back to the testing center). An assessor will flag an answer for the following reason:

"The response given indicates a dangerous, unethical, unprofessional or potentially harmful approach to the scenario that displays a clear deficiency in the candidate's ability to appreciate the complex ethical issues raised."

In the event that a response is flagged, the assessor is then obligated to comment on why they flagged the answer. The other reason assessors must elaborate on their flagging of an answer is to justify their reasons for flagging it. This mechanic acts as something of a fail-safe for a candidate's application process – the red-flagged response and the assessors' comments will be reviewed by an admissions officer or committee. If it is felt that the assessor was excessively harsh in their judgment of the response, and provided the remainder of the candidate's responses scored well, this red flag can be overlooked within the context of that candidate's overall application.

However, multiple red flags on a candidate's test score are likely to result in rejection of the application. You may be asking yourself, "What happens if my test is marked by an assessor with excessively high standards?" This is unlikely because importantly each scenario is marked by a different assessor making it very unlikely that you ended up with 12 assessors that were all difficult graders. Furthermore, given the instruction CASPer raters receive with regards to objective marking criteria, the marking system is set up to account for the possibility that some assessors have more critical approaches than others.

When marking CASPer, an assessor will usually be given a series of candidates' responses to the same scenario and questions. The claimed advantage in doing this is two-fold: the assessor can apply the same criteria to multiple applicants' responses rather than having to shift focus between subject matter every time AND the applicants have a different assessor marking each question rather than one continually harsh (or lenient) assessor for their whole test. This is claimed to be fairer and gives a more accurate representation of the candidates' interpersonal skills and ability to respond to the challenging scenarios CASPer presents.

Sample Questions, Answers and Discussions

As we mentioned before, practice is key when preparing for CASPer. As will be the case throughout your future medical career, a good way of learning new skills is by being shown how to do it first. This is particularly effective when applied to developing new psychomotor skills or physical procedures such as catheterization, intubation or any surgical procedure, but this approach can also be applied to cognitive reasoning skills and thought processing. The advantage of using this method in the latter is that you are able to learn how NOT to do things as well as how to do them – clearly professional ethical responsibilities prevent us from demonstrating how NOT to perform surgical procedures on real patients (though if you mess up using a training simulation model, it's not the end of your career!).

The following is a sample question just like the type you will encounter during CASPer. We will provide two responses for each question – an excellent response and a response likely to be red-flagged. We will then discuss why each response was good or bad and highlight what it was about the response that made them as such.

Question 1: You are a junior surgical resident scheduled to assist an attending surgeon in his operating room for his list that day. The attending surgeon arrives 20 minutes late and you notice he is stumbling around off-balance in the locker room while changing into scrubs and smells strongly of alcohol. How would you deal with this situation?

GOOD ANSWER: As a physician, my first duty of care is to the patient. If I felt that the attending surgeon was putting any patient at risk of harm at all, it would be my responsibility to alert another senior member of staff to the situation and enlist their help. Aside from alcohol consumption, in this situation, I should also be concerned whether or not the surgeon is a diabetic and experiencing an attack that makes him appear as though he is under the influence of alcohol. In either care, both for the safety of the patient and the surgeon, I would alert the appropriate hospital authorities to the surgeons' conduct.

BAD ANSWER: I would offer to make the surgeon some coffee before we began operating, as this would help him stay more awake and alert during surgery. If I saw that he was having difficulty with some parts of the procedures, I would offer to help or do those parts for him so we could finish on time.

DISCUSSION: It's clear from the stem that the attending surgeon is not fit to be operating. This has the potential to harm patients. This must absolutely be recognized – the first line of the Hippocratic Oath states that physicians shall "First, do no harm". Failure to acknowledge this is, at the very least, a low-scoring response. Although you are in the role of a junior in this situation, any physician must not allow a fellow physician to put patients at risk of serious harm by performing surgery while incapacitated, irrespective of seniority. That being said, in the interest of avoiding potential confrontation and conflict, seeking assistance in determining the surgeons' incapability of operating is a sensible and commendable course of action. To not only allow but facilitate the surgeon to operate in such a condition is negligence of the most serious sort and will more than likely result in medico-legal ramifications that would only be worsened if it transpired the resident performed part or all of the procedure that caused harm with inadequate supervision.

Follow-up question: In response to your suggestion that he cancels his operating list due to his condition, the attending surgeon angrily accuses you of insolence and threatens to have you removed from the residency program. How would you respond?

GOOD ANSWER: I would attempt to diffuse the situation by explaining my concern over possible patient harm and also express concern over the potential ramifications for the attending surgeon in the event that a patient was harmed. I would not directly acknowledge or address the threats as they are likely born out of the surgeon lashing out and may also be simply due to his medical condition. I would, however, stand my ground that I did not believe him to be in a fit state to perform surgery, and would be prepared to involve other members of staff who would likely concur with my assessment.

BAD ANSWER: I would back down and not raise the issue again. As the senior physician, he ultimately has more experience than I do and knows better when he is and is not fit to operate. I would also not make further comment at the risk of putting my job in jeopardy, since my family relies on my income alone and if I were to be fired as a result of this, it would effectively end my medical career.

DISCUSSION: The focus has now shifted from professional boundaries to conflict resolution – a classic scenario of a senior attempting to intimidate a junior colleague by threatening them. As before, the patient must come first. Even if you are having your career or job threatened by another physician, you cannot allow the patient to be exposed to a higher risk of serious injury. In reality, no medico-legal case against you can hope to be successful if you acted in the best interests of the patient, and it is also extremely unlikely that you will be removed from a residency program for doing so. Once again, introducing mediators or mitigation in the form of 3rd parties are invaluable approaches in resolving conflict, especially when they are likely to corroborate your assessment. Whilst you wouldn't necessarily be punished for doing so, backing down for fear of losing your job goes against the ethical principle of altruism and would certainly cost you marks in this type of scenario.

This type of question lends itself to group-style study as we previously mentioned. A good format for this would be to meet once a week (or as often as you like) for perhaps an hour or so in a group to discuss the scenario. Prior to the group session, one member of the group would be assigned to construct a "good" answer to the questions and another member would be assigned the task of writing a "bad" answer. The group would then discuss each answer after it has been presented and detail what made each answer good and bad. This strategy ensures that the group is well-versed in the ethical principles underling each scenario and is not only able to give a good response that includes consideration to said principles, but is also able to recognize when a response lacks the insight needed to score well on the test – knowing what NOT to do as well as what to do! But, as mentioned above, the best approach for preparing for the CASPer is doing realistic practice CASPer, such as those provided by BeMo's CASPer SIM™, and having your answers appraised by a trained professional.

It's also a good idea to run some of your mock responses by friends or family who have experience dealing with difficult ethical issues. Although medical professionals would be ideal, many walks of life deal with the types of situations you may encounter in the test, and the more people you consult, the more perspectives you gain. Being able to consider the issue from multiple sides is a favorable skill most assessors will recognize and reward.

Lastly, you should be aware that during your test, aside from scenario-based questions discussed above, you will also encounter personal type questions and policy type questions. Personal type questions are those that pertain to, or inquire about, your current and past experiences, values, belief systems, passions, etc. Personal type questions are those that are commonly encountered on a typical traditional panel interview. These include:

- *Describe a time when you came into a conflict with a peer or a colleague? How did you go about resolving it?*
- *Describe a time when you acted unprofessionally?*
- *What is your approach when dealing with an uncooperative group member?*

Alternatively, you can be provided a brief quotation or writing by an author and asked to reflect on the prose. This is yet another way of gaining insight into your personal characteristics.

It goes without saying that preparing for personal type questions is all about knowing yourself inside and out. It also helps to reflect on your past experiences and think about what qualities and characteristics were developed or refined and what lessons were learned during the experience. Specifically, when it comes to questions such as "describe a time when...,' which can be filled in with almost any scenario, it helps to structure your answer in the following manner.

Let's imagine you were asked to describe a time when you had a disagreement with a superior. The first thing you want to do is to provide a brief synopses or overview of the disagreement so that the reader can understand how the disagreement came about, who was involved, and what were the fundamental issues at play. You do not want to provide too much unrelated detail as this will eat up your time and space. Here is an example of a good synopses that allows you to set up the remainder of your answer:

"While I was a graduate student, my supervisor and I had an episode where we had different perspectives about how the collected data of our research study should be represented graphically and mathematically on a poster we were preparing for a presentation."

The above would be considered a clear and concise synopses of the disagreement and at this point you are ready to begin giving the most important part of the answer, which is how you went about resolving the conflict. It goes without saying that your approach to resolving disagreements should reflect your maturity and professionalism. Regardless of whether the disagreement is with a colleague, a peer, or a supervisor, you will need to be tactful and diplomatic. The following sample answer will shed more light on this matter:

"In trying to resolve our disagreement, I first set up a time where I could speak privately with my supervisor in hopes of having her explain her reasoning for the approach. I was fully aware that it could be my own lack of experience and insight that was leading to the disagreement and it was important for me to understand more about my supervisor's point of view prior to presenting my arguments. Once my supervisor presented her perspectives, I also shared mine and we were able to come to a new consensus about how to present the data."

The above would be considered a mature, professional and self-reflective answer. It also shows that you are capable of resolving disagreements in a tactful manner.

When dealing with policy type questions, where you are required to provide your opinion or views about a particular matter, there are a few things that you need to be aware of in order to be able to provide strong and appropriate responses. First of all, to be able to tackle policy type questions one needs to be very well read and up-to-date on the latest developments within the field of medicine. Having knowledge of current events and "hot-topic issues" such as physician-assisted suicide, medical marijuana, stem-cell research, etc. will also help in answering these types of questions.

In order to gain more information on the latest policies, current events, "hot-topic issues", and developments you will need to read the news on a daily basis, specifically the health and science sections. You can also learn more by visiting the American Medical Association's website (or the Canadian Medical Association for those in Canada) and your state or provincial association's website to stay current on the latest advancements and developments in the field of medicine.

One useful exercise in helping you learn more about current events and issues facing the healthcare system is to devise a top ten list of major issues. Once you have devised a list it will be time to begin doing some literature review and reading on the matter to see what the experts are saying about these issues and how they propose to resolve them. This way, if you come across a policy type question that asks you to discuss the number one concern facing the healthcare system and how you would propose to resolve it, you already have some talking points to draw upon. This type of policy question can also be asked in the following manner: Imagine you have been selected to provide the president with one policy to alter the American healthcare system. What one policy would you introduce and why? As you can see, once again, in order to be able to answer such a question, you will need to have done some background homework.

Now, when it comes to structuring your answer to a policy type question, we recommend that you first begin your answer with a short (one or two sentences) introduction that gives the reader an idea about your awareness of the issues and why such a policy would be discussed in the first place. Then, you will need to talk about the pros and cons associated with the policy and how they can negatively or positively impact the public, the patients, and lastly the doctors. This way your answer will not only be balanced and mindful of various perspectives, but it will more importantly be patient-centered rather than doctor-centered. What we mean by this is that if you begin talking about how the policy will positively and negatively affect the doctors prior to mentioning the public and the patients (the most important parties in the situation), your answer will be deemed too doctor-centered. You want to demonstrate that you will be a patient-centered future doctor.

Once you have presented both sides of the argument, then you can either take a stance on the matter or come up with an alternative solution to the issue proposed via the policy type question. Here is an example. Consider the following policy type question:

Currently, there are talks of implementing a 2-year mandatory work program for new medical graduates to be placed in rural and remote areas as part of their residency training. What are your views about such a policy?

Here is a sample answer, which entails all of the factors we discussed above. The answer will first start with a general introduction showing the writer's awareness of the issues. Then the pros and cons will be highlighted in a patient-centered manner, and lastly a unique solution will be provided.

"I understand the reasoning behind such a policy. There is currently a shortage of physician in remote settings and as such, this policy would attempt to remedy the problem. But of course, there are pros and cons involved. First, this policy would bring more doctors to underserved areas which is a great thing for those communities. The policy can also be beneficial as some doctors may end up staying in these communities long term. The experience will also enhance the skills of the doctors. However, this type of policy will create issues with continuity of care and the building of long-lasting and trusting relationships with the patient population. Unprepared candidates may also be forced to provide service and as a result of their lack of preparation they may cause more harm. And of course, we have to be mindful of the life demands of the doctors. This policy would be more ideal if it was voluntary. I do not agree with forcing candidates to enter such setting as the downsides could be costly to the population."

Final Thoughts

CASPer will require you to do lots of preparations in advance so that on test day you are comfortable with all of the obstacles that the test presents. Having presented you with all of the theoretical background in this chapter, which will hopefully help you to get started, you will now need to put theory into practice and take on some CASPer simulations to test your skills.

Summary – Top 10 CASPer Tips

1. Know your enemy – don't go into the exam unprepared or under-practiced

2. Practice honing your critical thinking and ethics skills well ahead of time
3. Do realistic CASPer simulations, with expert feedback
4. Read each question carefully
5. Take time to absorb & consider the situation, don't just write whatever comes to your head first
6. Don't rush your typing – answers that are hard to understand cost marks!
7. If you get mixed up, go back to your framework
8. If you slip up on a question or run out of time, just move on
9. Re-read your responses if you have the time
10. Remember – "First, do no harm"

For additional tips, sample videos, and questions, visit BeMo's online resource center for CASPer at https://caspertestprep.com/

CHAPTER VII

Admissions Interviews – Preparation Strategies & Winning Mindset

You've made the effort to perform well in school and on the MCAT. You've invested the time in your extracurricular activities to develop strong non-cognitive skills. You've prepared for and crushed CASPer. You've built relationships with referees who will encourage schools to accept you. You've gone to the expense of time and money to fill out applications. You've crafted an engaging personal statement and demonstrated further evidence of your suitability for medical school in you supplemental or secondary applications. But it's still not over. The last step before your acceptance is to attend an interview and astound a medical school with your communication skills and professionalism!

You might be asking why an interview is so important – or even why is an interview used at all. Doesn't an activities sketch already demonstrate non-cognitive skill development? How come a transcript doesn't let schools know how an applicant thinks? Shouldn't a personal statement already give schools an impression of the individual applicant? Why don't references speak to an applicant's character and suitability for medicine? Unfortunately, no component of an application is perfect. Having several means of assessment spreads out the "imperfection" allowing medical schools the opportunity to make sure you are the right fit for their program and the practice of medicine. While interviews may have some flaws, they are actually the best predictor of how you will perform as a future medical student at the time of writing this book. They are the most accurate means of assessing your ability to deal with challenging and complex situations and work with other people. Moreover, interviews are face-to-face and thus allow medical schools to better verify the skills and qualities you described on your paper application. The format also allows medical schools to assess how you put these skills and qualities into action in real-life scenarios. Further, interviews allow medical schools to see skills that cannot be shown on paper, including how you behave under pressure and the first impression you make. This is why your performance during the interview is a big factor in whether or not you are admitted to medical school. Often, it's the most significant portion of your entire application.

You could be interviewed by anyone who has a vested interest in your admission. This could include a member of the public because he/she may be your patient one day. It may also be a nurse, pharmacist, chiropractor, or other members of the allied healthcare team because they will be your future teammate. You could be questioned by a current medical student because you will be his/her classmate next year. Perhaps a resident or staff physician will speak with you because she will be your supervisor and teacher in the future. Because each member of this diverse group shares their own perspective of you, medical schools have a better idea of the effect you have on the people you'll encounter in medical school and how you will perform in the classroom and clinical area.

You might not know the role of your interviewer, but all assessors evaluate you on the same things. Questions are scored on three parameters. First, the effectiveness and appropriateness of your response. Second, the communication skills you used in expressing your thoughts. Third, your suitability for the medical profession. This last point can seem extremely subjective. Your suitability for medicine is determined by the professional skills and qualities that you convey through your responses. Again, one of the objectives of the interview is to allow the interviewer to form an impression of you as a medical student and future physician. How easily an interviewer is able to do this depends not only on the content of your responses and communication skills, but your non-verbal communication skills, ability to build rapport with an interviewer, confidence, and ability to perform under pressure.

You may hear that there are no right or wrong answers to interview questions. That's not entirely wrong but it isn't completely accurate. There are no right or wrong answers because, as you can see, you're scored on how you respond and the impression that you provide the interviewer. You can feel free to respond honestly without worry that assessors are looking for specific answers or marking you on particular statements. However, while there are no right or wrong answers there are certainly good and bad answers and appropriate and inappropriate responses. You will score poorly if you provide a bad answer. This could be an answer that is either lacking in content, communication skills or maturity of thought. Answers that are unprofessional or disrespectful are inappropriate answers. Instead of scoring poorly on a single question, these types of responses will jeopardize your entire application.

As with all elements of your application, preparing for an interview requires a great deal of work. Because interviews are so helpful in distinguishing between the quality of applicants, interview scores make up a sizable portion of your entire application. Admission statistics show that even individuals with above-average GPA and MCAT scores won't be admitted if they perform poorly, while those who may have a lower than average academic record can gain entry if they do well in the interview. **This means you can think of the interview like a gatekeeper for medical school**. In an extremely competitive process where so few people are admitted, you give yourself the best chance for success by devoting the necessary time to practice.

One of the first steps in preparing for your interview is determining the type of interview you'll have. This will give you a framework for your practice because you'll be able to prepare for the structure of the interview and the types of questions being asked.

The Multiple Mini Interview (MMI)

The MMI is becoming an increasingly common method of interviewing. Unlike traditional interviews where you would be asked questions by the same interviewer(s) in series, MMIs are between eight to twelve separate "stations" where you are assessed by individual interviewers (typically, there are one or two break stations included for rest). The rationale behind this structure is to decrease assessor bias by having multiple interviewers. This format is also to the advantage of the applicant; if you perform poorly on one station, it does not affect the impression other interviewers may hold of you. Each station will be between four and eight minutes. You'll be outside your interview room and given a brief amount of time to read your prompt, which will be posted outside the door. After your time to review the prompt has elapsed, you'll be instructed to enter the interview room and begin interacting with your interviewer. You will be given a longer time to answer your question, but this will be very brief. This is why it is essential to practice in realistic conditions because simulations will help you adapt to the time pressure and develop skills in forming concise responses. After your interview time has elapsed, you will be instructed to leave the room and go to your next station where another prompt will be posted outside the door.

You can expect to encounter a mix of question types among all the stations. Most commonly, scenario based questions and competency/skills based questions are used more heavily, followed by policy-type questions. There are usually one or two interacting and task-based questions; behavioral questions may or may not be included. You will likely NOT encounter any knowledge-based scenarios (i.e. specific medical ethical questions, scenarios requiring medical knowledge); remember, the MMI is designed to test non-cognitive skills and is looking for the ideal medical student, they don't expect you to already have the knowledge that you will learn in medical school.

Before we move on to the other interview formats, it is important to note here that, although there has been some research pointing to the efficacy of multiple mini interviews as an admissions tool, the majority of such research has been done by the same researchers/university that have now turned this interview format into a for-profit company and, in our opinion, such claims must be viewed with caution until further independent studies have been conducted to verify multiple mini interview's validity and efficacy or until the MMI is replaced by a better and more reliable admissions tool.

Panel Interview

Even though the MMI is claimed to reduce bias and assessor error in interviews, applicants can still prepare and perform well in panel interviews. In panel interviews, you'll be interviewed by a group of assessors who will each take turns asking questions in series. Your responses will be evaluated by the group and each individual's overall impression of your performance will form the basis of your score. Therefore, it's important to keep focused and clearheaded so that you can form the best impression you can on all of your panel members. The duration of a panel interview is usually provided to you before you attend. If not, you should request this information from the school. Typically, panel interviews can last anywhere from twenty minutes to a full hour.

Panel interviews include some of the types of questions that you can expect on an MMI, including policy type or scenario based questions. Even though the structure of the interview is different, your approach to answering these types of questions is the same between the two interviews. Panel interviews also include more personal questions, quirky questions, and personal type questions based off your application. It would be quite unusual for panel interviews to include a task-based or interaction-based questions.

Modified Panel Interview (MPI)

MPI is a new interview format first introduced by the University of Toronto's medical program. The initial reason for the introduction of MPIs was to ensure that traditional interviews, which are known to be ineffective tools, are no longer used and further, to match the supposed reliability and validity of MMIs without all of the resource expenditure. Although an MPI, like many interviews strives to assess interpersonal qualities, an MPI is different than an MMI and a traditional Panel. An MPI allows a candidate to be interviewed separately by four distinct individuals. These individuals, all of whom have had the opportunity to read over the candidate's application, can be a faculty member, a student, healthcare professional etc. On the day of the interview, the candidate will move from room to room carrying out each interview, typically lasting from 10-12 minutes. The types of questions encountered during a MPI are typically behavioral questions, personal and school specific questions that are related to the healthcare system, scenario-based questions, and questions that come with a twist. For example, "teach me something most people cannot do" would be considered a quirky question with a twist. The candidates are rated among three common attributes: maturity, communication skills, and interpersonal skills, and a fourth attribute unique to the interviewees.

Hybrid Interviews
You can think of a hybrid interview as a mix of the MMI and the panel interview. This usually looks like a smaller version of a typical MMI (meaning fewer stations although the length of time and format of the stations are the same) combined with a shorter panel or individual interview. There is a lot of diversity between schools on how each hybrid interview is run and you should ask each school the times used for the MMI and other interview portion. You can expect the same questions on a typical MMI to appear in your MMI section of the interview. Likewise, you can expect typical panel-style questions for your panel or individual interview section. This will require you to prepare for scenario-based questions, policy-type questions, competency/skills based questions, personal type questions, quirky type questions, and personal type questions based on your application.

Preparation Tips and Tricks

1) Do your homework
There is no way around it! You have to prepare for the interview. If you come unprepared, interviewers will worry that you will be unprepared for medical school. Take the task seriously. Make sure you practice and have a good grasp of topics you may potentially be asked. You should have a good command of issues that are common themes for interview questions. Keep up to date with current events. Read the news. Review medical ethics and reasoning. Become aware of issues important to the general public and those relevant for healthcare. This is an abbreviated list but it will help you get started:

a) Social determinants of health
b) Rural and urban health disparities
c) End-of-life care
d) Mental health care
e) Racialized violence
f) Healthcare reform
g) Childhood vaccinations

2) *Perfect* practice makes perfect

You might be more familiar with "practice makes perfect". In reality, most applicants are far from perfect when they practice especially when they first begin. Continuing to practice this way only reinforces habits that won't serve you well in your actual interview. This means that you want to practice in simulated conditions that best resemble conditions on your interview day. Not only will the quality of your practice improve, but you'll feel more comfortable and familiar with the environment on interview day. Make sure that you receive objective feedback on your performance from interview professionals so you can identify your mistakes and learn from them. You will likely find many people who are invested in your success and have good intentions, but only those who are familiar with the interview process and scoring interview questions will help you develop effective responses. These include any healthcare professionals (NOT medical students) who have been on interview committees. If you don't have anyone to help you, invest in yourself and take advantage of BeMo's interview prep programs.

3) Don't forget non-verbal communication

A huge portion of the impression that you will make on your interviewer comes from the things that you don't actually say. Research shows that 90% of communication is non-verbal communication! Dress professionally. Smile and maintain eye contact. Greet your interviewer. Sit comfortably in your chair without fidgeting or slouching. Keep both feet on the floor. Many of these things go beyond simple courtesies or social vanities and form the opinion the public holds of physicians. Include these in your practice so you are well used to them by interview time. An added benefit to practicing in your interview clothes is that you won't find out your shoes don't fit or there is a stain on your shirt on one of the biggest days of your life!

4) Don't forget to reflect

With all the emphasis on what impression you give your interviewers, it's easy to overlook your role in the process too. An important piece of your preparation is self-reflection. This is helpful in a number of ways. If you're self-aware you'll be able to identify your weaknesses in interview practice and target your preparation more effectively. As well, you'll have a clearer view of your application to draw from your experience and provide stronger examples of the skills you developed. Lastly, reflect on why you want to be a physician and why the application process is worth it for you. This is a stressful, time consuming, and expensive endeavor. You should know for sure that it is what you want to pursue and be able to express why that is.

5) Manage your anxiety

It's understandable how nerves could get the best of anyone. This is one of the most important steps in the interview process. It's highly competitive. It may be your first time having an official medical school interview. There's an immense time pressure. The list of reasons to be stressed is long – but it's not as long as the list of reasons why it's important to do well. Your goal is to be a physician and you've worked hard to get to this point. Forgive yourself for maybe having a poor night's sleep or a few butterflies in your stomach, but don't stand in your own way.

6) Remember that you are choosing them as much as they are choosing you!

Most students walk into the interview room with the mindset that they must be on their best behavior (rather than being themselves) to impress the school's officers and interviewers. But you must realize that your job at an interview also includes getting a better sense of the program including their visions and long-term mission. If you have done your homework you should feel confident that you are a good candidate and that you are choosing med schools as much as they are choosing you. This is an important mindset and it will shift the balance of power in your favor and helps you remain confident. Think about it, what if you go for your interview and you find out that the medical school's missions and long-term visions are contradictory to yours? Would you still want to go and help them with their cause if you have options? (And if you do everything we talk about in this book, you will certainly have options!)

Stress Management

There is an undeniable connection between your mind and body. If you feel nervous and anxious, you'll show visible signs of stress. Similarly, you can take cues from your behavior to identify when you need to get your nerves under control. If you hear your voice waver, feel your shoulders tense, or find yourself fidgeting in your chair take a deep and slow breath. Deep breathing (take a few seconds to inhale and then slowly exhale) helps turn off your "fight or flight" stress reaction and stimulates relaxation. Your body will respond by decreasing the amount of stress hormones you produce, reducing your heart rate and you'll be able to think more clearly. You'll not only feel more relaxed, but you'll appear more comfortable and show interviewers that you're in command of your emotions and confident in your performance. This will help your communication skills and, as you do better in the interview, you'll feel more comfortable. You can continue deep breathing exercises on your interview day by beginning each station (or before entering the interview room) with a deep breath. Not only will you enter the station feeling more at ease, but this will also give you a needed pause so you don't rush your answer. Throughout the application process, make sure you are taking good care of yourself. You'll be better able to cope with any stressful situation if you are in good health mentally and physically. Make sure you are exercising regularly, eating nutritiously, and sleeping as much as you can. Take time to decompress by doing stress-relieving activities you enjoy. Focusing on your overall wellness as you prepare for interviews doesn't seem like a priority but you won't believe the difference it can make.

There are also other strategies you can use to manage stress in the weeks and months leading up to your interview and on the actual day. Don't underestimate the value of practice for relieving stress. It's easy to feel overwhelmed and delay practicing, but procrastinating only makes things worse. If you feel prepared and know that you have done all you can to set yourself up for success you will eliminate a lot of unnecessary worry. Practicing with realistic simulations and receiving professional advice is also important in helping you feel at ease on your interview day. Although medical students are not an appropriate resource for interview guidance since they are by definition still going through their training, you can speak with current medical students to get a better idea of what to expect and gain insight into the atmosphere of the interviews. Make sure that you find out where to go for interviews before the actual interview day. You should definitely know the correct location and the amount of time that it will take to get there. Running behind in time or getting lost are two of the easiest but most anxiety provoking problems to solve. Additionally, you should visit the building, walk around, read a book on location, and even have a meal there a few days before you interview. This is to eliminate the fear of the unknown, at least when it comes to the interview location.

By the time interview day arrives, you should have done all the preparation that you need to do. You shouldn't feel the need to practice on the day before your interview. Use this time to put yourself at ease by doing activities that you enjoy. Continue to keep your stress relieving habits of exercising, eating well and sleeping adequate hours a priority. Remember the mind-body connection and use this to your advantage. Smiling has a similar effect on stress relief as deep breathing and you'll appear more warm and welcoming to your interviewers. Assuming a confident body posture will decrease the visible signs of stress and help interviewers picture you as being confident as a physician more easily. Consider finding ways to identify and manage stress as it is as important as your actual practice for interviews and your investment in coping with the anxiety of interviews will pay off immensely.

Now that you're familiar with the different types of medical school interviews, you can begin familiarizing yourself with the types of questions you might encounter during these sessions.

Different types of interview questions and stations

Situational/scenario based stations

These are the most commonly asked questions in Multiple Mini Interviews. In these questions, you will be provided with a prompt about a real-life scenario and given a role within the situation and then asked to discuss your approach for dealing with the situation at hand. You might be asked what you would do in a given situation and how you would respond to another person in the prompt. Occasionally you may be asked a probing question where one of the variables in the prompt is changed. Many applicants will focus their preparation for scenario-based questions on medical ethics and the professional qualities of physicians. Usually, applicants don't apply these to non-clinical questions and rely on their individual reasoning. Discussing real-life scenarios with applicants allows medical schools to determine if you actually have good judgment or if you are simply applying your interview preparation to other scenarios. Keep in mind that, although these scenarios don't appear to be medically related, the non-cognitive skills that are being assessed are transferable to situations you'll encounter as a medical student and throughout your career as a physician. For this reason, you should keep your medical ethics in mind when answering these questions and make sure your response reflects the emotional intelligence that would be expected of a physician. Here is a sample scenario-based question:

Your friend Jamie has flown across the country to visit her family. Before traveling, Jamie left her car keys with you so that you could pick her up from the airport when she gets back. You don't have a car of your own so you were appreciative that she lent hers to you. She chose you for this task because she doesn't want anyone else driving her car and has asked you not to let anyone else use it. The last time she left town, one of her friends took a passenger to a sports game and left mud all over the seats! She made it clear that only you are allowed to use the car.

Jamie's family time is very important to her as she rarely gets to see them. She's told you that she has turned her phone off and has asked you not to get in contact with her by other means for any reason throughout her holiday.

The day after Jamie left, your friend Marnie called. You were busy and missed her but heard this when you checked your voicemail:

> *"Hi! It's Marnie! I know that Jamie left her car keys with you and I was hoping you could do me a big favor. The store where I work is having a big shipment come in tomorrow. I'm supposed to pick it up but my car broke down. Can you lend me the keys to pick it up? Or maybe drive me yourself? I wouldn't ask if it wasn't really important. I'm worried I will be fired if I don't get this shipment. Please help!"*

Here is a sample answer (after you take a deep breath, smile, and greet your interviewer!):

> *"As I understand, I have two very good friends who have asked for my help. My friend, Jamie, has asked me to take care of her car and has set clear rules that only I may use it. My friend, Marnie, really needs a vehicle for work and would like to use Jamie's car. Unfortunately, I can't contact Jamie for her thoughts. I have to consider my duty to Jamie and how I can help Marnie. I think I would first reflect on the challenge that is before me. I want to keep Jamie's trust. However, I also value Marnie's friendship and I don't want to avoid helping her, particularly because I can imagine she feels an extraordinary amount of pressure at work and fears losing her job. With that in mind, I would call Marnie back as soon as possible because I need to address this with her promptly. I would ask her what type of shipment it is and why she is so fearful about losing her position. I would also want to know if she was aware of the rules that Jamie had for using her car. I wouldn't make any assumptions that Marnie is disregarding Jamie's wishes and I also wouldn't let the fact that Jamie might not find out cloud my judgment. Then, I would explain to her that*

I couldn't use Jamie's car for this because she's asked me not to and I have to respect her wishes. I want Marnie to know that by doing what Jamie has asked of me, Marnie can also have trust that I'll do what she might ask me to do in the future. How can she trust me to follow through on what I tell her if I break Jamie's confidence now? That being said, I also want Marnie to know that I understand that she is in a very challenging position and I want to help her. I would offer solutions, like asking another friend to borrow a car, or suggest using a rental or taxi service. If it doesn't seem like Marnie will be able to pick up the shipment for work, I would offer suggestions on how she could communicate this to her boss and provide assistance so she doesn't feel so overwhelmed with that task. I think this is the best course of action because I can still be of assistance to Marnie and follow Jamie's direction."

Approach to scenario-based questions

Remember that these are real-life scenarios that can be transferred to clinical situations. Imagine if Jamie was a patient of yours who shared personal information and Marnie was another patient who was asking what Jamie had told you. Whether or not that information is helpful to Marnie is irrelevant. You have a duty to protect Jamie's confidentiality. If you broke confidentiality with Jamie, you would also break any future trust with Marnie. Using medical ethics in this situation makes the answer clearer and this intuition will develop with practice. First, make sure to read the prompt slowly so you understand the situation and can identify the type of scenario you've been given. The example above is a scenario that assesses trustworthiness. Next, you'll want to gather as much information as you can; make sure you explain what else you need to know and what questions you would ask. Don't rush to make any conclusions or snap decisions: be clear that you want to be non-judgmental. After doing this, you should identify the most pressing issues in your scenario. In this prompt, the main challenge was helping Marnie while still following Jamie's rules. Identifying these issues correctly allows you to offer practical solutions and suggestions. You can conclude scenario-based questions by choosing a logical and ethical course of action and describing how your decision affects the people directly or indirectly involved.

Interacting (i.e.: role play, debate with partner) station

These stations are designed to test your communication, collaboration, and teamwork skills. You will be partnered with your interviewer or, more commonly, another applicant to complete a task. You might be asked to role play in a scenario, debate a topical issue, or create or build an item together. These types of stations can mislead you to think you will score highly if you outshine your partner or promptly find a solution to the problem that you've been given. It's still important that you perform well, but by maintaining clear and respectful communication you will actually be able to do this. Just as importantly, you will show that you can successfully work with others even under pressure and time constraints. Here is a sample question:

You are neighbors with an elderly couple, Frank and Diane, who have always been good friends to you and your family. Sadly, Diane passed away last year after a long illness. You and your family, but especially Frank, miss her very much. Over the past few months, you've noticed that Frank has not seemed the same. The house that was once neat and tidy now has an overgrown yard and chipped paint. Calls to Frank go unreturned. When you see him come out of the house, his clothes are dirty and his hair is messy. Some of the other neighbors are worried that Frank continues to drive and is dangerous in his current state of mind. Because of your close relationship with Frank, you have been asked to speak with him about his driving. When you enter the room, you will be meeting with Frank to discuss this.

Approach to this station

When you enter the room, you will see an assessor and an actor who will obviously be Frank. Interviewers are generally quite fair in helping you figure out who is the assessor and who is the actor; you won't need to worry about who to speak with. In acting stations, it's generally best to say a brief hello to the assessor before turning your attention fully to the actor. Otherwise, the initial approach to these types of questions is similar to other questions. Just like you would greet an assessor and recap your prompt, you will greet Frank and provide details as to why you're meeting before beginning a discussion. A successful approach is to show that you are empathetic and non-judgmental, but can still recognize when action needs to be taken.

After you say hello and ask how Frank is, you can lead into your discussion by saying, "I always enjoyed our social visits Frank, but today I've come to talk about something difficult. I want to let you know there have been some concerns raised about your safety on the road and I wanted to get your perspective. Do you have any concerns about your driving?" It's important that Frank understands that you want to discuss road safety, but also that you require his side of the story; right now you are only acting on others' concerns. While you have observed a change in his personality, this could be a sign of many things, including depression, dementia, mourning, or poor health, and you want to be able to help him as best you are able. You can explain the situation further by saying, "I know you've had an incredibly difficult time this past year without Diane. When anyone experiences a loss like that, it takes some time before they feel like themselves again. But sometimes people are affected by something other than grief. Do you feel safe driving and safe in your home?" Further, you can introduce the additional content in the prompt by saying "It's completely understandable that you haven't been able to spend the same amount of time on yard work and laundry. Can you tell me if anything has been particularly overwhelming?" It's important to show empathy for the challenges he's faced and acknowledge that you may have to intervene. Most often, applicants do this by saying something like "That sounds really tough" or "That must be hard for you." These phrases sound trite and insincere because they are used so frequently. Try to use more original phrases like, "It seem like this has really affected you negatively" or "I can see how sad you are about this." You'll also demonstrate empathy more effectively when paraphrasing what the actor has told you. For example, "What I'm hearing you say is that you've been so lonely it's hard to think about anything else."

Asking non-judgmental questions is the best way to gather information to help you propose solutions. You will begin to get an inclination on what you can offer Frank based on his answers. You may find that he just needs some extra support at home so you could offer to help him around the house or drive for him. Maybe he is still grieving from Diane's death and you tell him that you are able to help him any way you can and suggest a counselor. It could be that he has begun to notice his health failing and so you could suggest that you take him to his physician's office for an assessment. Perhaps you are more certain that he has a serious cognitive disability and propose taking him to his doctor for more urgent help.

The solutions that you provide should reflect your empathy and your practicality. An easy mistake to make is to believe that assessors are looking for the biggest gestures of generosity and the largest amount of suggestions. Your suggestions should show that you are realistic and able to maintain appropriate boundaries. Don't "over-promise" or step out of your role in the scenario. For example, it might seem to be a very compassionate response to offer Frank to move into your home and care for him, but very few neighbors would actually do this. Try to resist the urge to go above and beyond what would normally expected of someone in your scenario even if you're not sure what to offer or say. "I wish I knew what I could do to help; I'm happy to just listen if you want to talk more," shows more insight and better judgment than unrealistic propositions. This shows that not only can you provide help to your future patients and colleagues if you are called upon, you will be aware of your own limitations and maintain professional boundaries.

Here is another sample interaction station question (i.e. debate question):

The influenza virus can cause an unpleasant but ultimately harmless and relatively brief sickness. However, for the very young and very old, pregnant women, and frail and chronically ill individuals, the flu can have serious health risks including death. At present, there are only a few jurisdictions where the flu vaccination is mandatory for healthcare workers; those who do not wish to have the vaccine must wear a mask while at work. This policy was instituted because healthcare workers are at high risk for contracting the flu virus, and thus it can save employers valuable sick time. As well, it would help avoid transmission to at-risk patients. However, this policy has come under fire for infringing on workers' rights to self-determination. Because they are forced to identify themselves as being unvaccinated by means of having a mask, workers may also have their personal choices made public and questioned. You will be asked to debate this policy with a partner.

Applicant A, you will be arguing in favor of this policy.

Applicant B, you will be arguing against this policy.

Approach to this station

These stations are those where applicants especially feel the need to compete with their fellow debater, who is most often an applicant as well. Instead of imagining yourself in competition, imagine yourself in a classroom with a peer who made a statement with which you disagree. In that situation, you can perform brilliantly if you can acknowledge any validity in your classmate's opinion while diplomatically explaining why you disagree and providing a logical counter argument. Are you respectful of people, even if you don't share the same views? Do you stay true to your beliefs even if told otherwise? Can you find a realistic compromise when presented challenging issues? These are some of the questions assessors will be asking during your debate. It's reassuring to know that you can prepare a significant knowledge base for these types of stations simply by preparing for the interview in general. Essentially, these are scenario-based or policy-type questions that also assess communication and collaboration.

Try to focus on making between one to three well-developed points. Of course you can make more arguments if you feel you are able, but it's more likely that the time constraints will be such that you can only provide a minimum quantity of points to ensure maximum quality. Make sure you justify your arguments and provide your reasoning. For example, "As the prompt alluded to, mandatory flu vaccines can prevent sick time and the transmission of the virus to patients. This will ensure that there are no unnecessary healthcare costs for personnel or staff shortages that negatively impact patient care. Patients have a reasonable expectation of their healthcare providers that they have their best interests at heart. Patients wouldn't feel safe seeking care from healthcare providers who might transmit a virus with the potential of a serious illness or death. Further, it would be against the ethical duty of clinicians to put their patients at risk. It would be wrong to create an environment where patients who need help face a personal risk to receive that help. Avoiding the vaccine but still wearing a mask allows clinicians their autonomy while still protecting patients' rights. An additional point I would like to add is that mandating vaccines for healthcare providers sends a message to the public about their safety and efficacy and could encourage others to get the flu vaccine for themselves. This would give them the personal benefit of preventing the flu as well as broader benefits to the community."

When it is your turn to rebut your partner's argument, it's important to start off on a collegial tone that demonstrates you have considered his or her point of view. You can then offer why you feel his or her argument is incorrect before continuing on to make your own points. "Thank you for your thoughts. You are certainly correct that it would be very beneficial if healthcare workers did not contract the flu virus and your point that it would encourage others to be more proactive about their own health is very well taken. However, in my opinion, your arguments are all on the condition that the correct strains of influenza have been identified and the vaccine has been administered before any exposure occurs. I'm not sure that's always possible and I think it would be wrong to impose on healthcare providers' rights to choose their own healthcare with that uncertainty. Most clinicians do not want to harm their patients, even if they don't want to be vaccinated. This may be why they choose to practice good hand hygiene, which is an effective way to prevent transmission of the flu and other infectious disease." Your argument must be clear and valid, but you will stand out in this station by being respectful and diplomatic.

Task-based question (i.e.: drawing or building an object)

Just as in interacting stations, task-based stations also test your communication and team building skills. However, these stations allow interviewers to see how you behave when giving and receiving instructions. Imagine that you are a physician counseling a patient who has high blood pressure. The objective of your appointment will be to prescribe an anti-hypertensive.

You might think that you have completed your task when you have written the prescription, but no patient is going to take a medication unless they understand what it is for and why it is important. Similarly, imagine you are in a drawing station. Your task will be to either complete the drawing yourself or instruct your partner to finish the illustration. Assessors will be looking for how clearly you ask questions and give responses and how easily you build rapport with your partner before they assess the drawing you re-created. The focus of your assessment then, will be on how you communicate. It's important that you can be productive and can achieve your objectives, even under pressure, but the main indicator of your performance will be how you communicate with your partner. There is an immense amount of teaching required to help a novice student gain proficiency and competency throughout medical school. How receptive are you to instructions and feedback? Can you follow through on tasks? Do you ask for help or clarification when needed? These questions need to be answered, and are utilized by medical schools to assess your abilities before deciding whether or not they want to invest the time to teach you. While you may not know much at the start, your ability to thrive on challenge, and better yourself will still be evaluated. Now keep in mind, you will learn a great deal throughout your training. You'll gain enough expertise that you will be able to counsel your patients, instruct medical students and residents, and pass on information to your colleagues. However, at the end of the day, medical schools need to know that you feel comfortable asking questions, provide concise explanations, and essentially understand complicated material and tasks.

Example of drawing station

Applicant A: You have been given an illustration that your partner has never seen before. Please provide instructions to your partner so that he or she can recreate the drawing.

Applicant B: You have been given a blank piece of paper and a pencil. Your partner has an image that he or she will describe for you. Please follow these directions to recreate the drawing using the supplies you have been given.

Approach to task based questions

These types of questions are also similar to interacting stations because of the temptation to outshine your fellow applicant. In reality, being clear, calm, and focused will make you stand out. Don't forget that these stations also have the same requirements as any other station. Greet your interviewer and your partner and clarify the task you have been given. For example, a statement like, "Let's make sure we're on the same page. You have a drawing and I have a blank page. You've been asked to give me some instructions and I've been asked to follow them to draw the picture you have," shows that you're able to identify a common goal. Healthcare is becoming increasingly team-based and it's important that all members of the team understand their role and what they aim to achieve as individuals and as a group. If you're in the role of providing instructions be as clear and simple as you possibly can. Imagine yourself giving instructions to a patient who doesn't have any medical knowledge. For example, describing a shape as round instead of using the word spherical is a far more effective way of communicating in these stations. Don't forget to include detail in your descriptions because this minimizes the chance of miscommunication. Think of how your partner would draw a circle if you told him or her "Draw a circle" compared to if you said, "I'm looking at my paper widthwise and there is a circle with a four centimeter diameter centered in the page. Can you please draw that for yourself and let me know when you are done?" It's important to show that you can give direction and provide instruction, but also that you do so in a respectful way that doesn't make others feel subservient or patronized. If your partner asks a question or doesn't seem to understand, use different wording instead of repeating the same explanations. Avoid the urge to start your instructions with things like "Now you will," or "I want you to." Furthermore, give your partner ample time and ask if he or she has any questions or would like to re-evaluate how instructions are given. When you pause to ask "Can you let me know what you have drawn so far?" or "How is this working for you? Is there anything that you think would make this task easier?" you show that you haven't lost sight of the fact that this is as much a team-based station as it is task-based. If you are receiving the instructions to complete the task, make sure that you are also engaged in the station. Let your partner know when you have finished a step and ask questions as you need. Take opportunities to provide feedback on how things are going. You can, for example, say things such as, "I'll take a minute to tell you what I've drawn to make sure we are going down the right path. When we restart, I'd really appreciate it if you could slow down your instructions. I am having a hard time keeping up and don't want to miss anything."

Imagine yourself in a learning scenario as a future medical student. Assessors want to know that you can take ownership of your learning, ask for help when it is needed, and are focused and attentive to directions. Ultimately, the most successful applicants at these stations – whether giving or receiving instructions – are those who work best together.

Policy type questions

Policy type questions will introduce a topic and assess your understanding of the issue and your awareness of different perspectives on the matter. You might be asked to state the pros, cons, and alternatives to a particular policy. More commonly, applicants are asked how they feel about a certain topic and if they agree or disagree. On the surface, these stations assess your knowledge of topics that may be important politically, economically, or socially and thus, have implications on patients and the healthcare they receive. However, they also assess emotional intelligence. Policy type questions can give medical schools a small window into your personal belief system. Do you understand and respect others' rights? Do you believe in fulfilling duties and responsibilities? Can you recognize when right and wrong are black and white and when they are ambiguous? What do you value when deciding whether or not to support a particular policy? What do you consider when deciding whether or not something is right or wrong? In these stations you want to demonstrate that you try to learn as much as you can about an issue and consider all perspectives before making a judgment. As well, you want to demonstrate good moral reasoning and highlight that you stay true to what you believe is right.

Example of policy type question

Many medical students feel overwhelmed and overworked with their responsibilities as learners. One of these responsibilities is to be present in the hospital while on-call and the length of these shifts is thought to contribute to sleeplessness and stress. Because of concerns for medical students' wellness, some schools have transitioned from the traditional 24-hour call shift model to a 16-hour model. Opponents of this policy argue that increasing the time away from clinical duties removes medical students from important learning experiences during formative years of their training. This might result in decreased preparation for the next stages of their training. Do you believe medical students should be working 24- or 16-hour call shifts?

Approach to policy type questions

Fortunately, it is not hard to demonstrate positive qualities and emotional intelligence in these stations if you have a good approach. The most important part of your response is the completion of your answer. This means that you do not simply provide your opinion. If you only provide how you feel about a policy, you will fail to demonstrate any non-cognitive skills or that you have the capacity to gather information and consider the opinions of others involved. First, acknowledge the complexity of the issue and state why you think a policy like this may be needed. This will demonstrate that you have an awareness of the issue. Second, you should take the time to explain why you feel others agree or disagree (essentially, a list of pros and cons) with the policy. By examining different perspectives, you demonstrate that you recognize all sides of an issue must be considered before making a decision. After this, you can state your own beliefs and opinion on the policy.

Even though you've already provided a list of pros and cons, you want to make sure to include the rationale for your decision. Using this approach will make sure that your response is organized and easy to follow. More importantly, it will allow you to demonstrate the important skills and qualities necessary to deal with issues in the healthcare system in the future. It may be possible that you can find a compromise or propose an alternative solution to a policy. If so, you should include it in your answer. Don't forget that you must always answer what a station asks of you. If it asks for your opinion, you are best to offer it as well.

Policies in hospitals, professional organizations, and provinces and countries affect the day-to-day work of physicians. Medical schools need to know that you have the maturity and thoughtfulness to work under these policies and maintain a strong code of ethics.

Sample answer: (Again, don't forget to take a deep breath and greet your interviewer!)

"The task I've been given is to discuss the implementation of shorter on-call time requirements for medical students. I know that this policy deals with issues much more complex than simply the hours that medical students work. The call policy balances students' need for rest with the opportunities in their learning environment. I think it's important to have a policy on call shift times to make sure that the demands of medical school do not come at an expense of students' personal wellness. But, it's also important to make sure that such a policy doesn't limit their learning opportunities or decrease the quality of their training and preparation for the future. I can see how people could be divided on this issue.

To be on call for 24-hours is extremely demanding. For those who have to balance learning and adjusting to a new professional role, 24 hour on-call shifts can be extremely demanding. If medical students are overtired, the quality of their learning will decrease irrespective of their exposure. Further, overworking medical students puts patients at risk because of the potential for errors in patient-care as a result of mental fatigue. It also endangers students because they may not be safe to drive themselves home. Those who don't agree with the policy make a strong argument as well.

Simply decreasing call shift times is not enough to reduce student fatigue because there are many more reasons why a rigorous program would be stressful. There are likely other measures, like mentoring partnerships and wellness programs, that will improve student health without decreasing their exposure to important learning opportunities. Some people think it's important that medical students don't miss the eight hours that this policy takes away because in those eight hours they will see more patients, participate in more care, and, thus, be able to provide better care in the future. And, perhaps by being exposed to more situations, students will feel more prepared and less stressed for their call shifts and school in general.

After looking at both sides of the issue, I personally believe that there may be a compromise. An effective policy would be one where students rotating through the busiest areas have 16-hour call days and students assigned to less busy areas work 24-hour call days. The students working in busy areas still get their exposure to learning opportunities while still being able to rest and have more personal time. The students in the less busy areas will likely have more rest on their call shift and better able to stay for 24-hours without otherwise losing out on important learning experiences."

Or alternatively, the answer you provide could take on a side and be less compromising than the one shown above. For instance,

"When I consider both sides of this issue, I find that I side with those who are in favor of decreasing the length of call shifts for medical students. I think it's a reasonable argument that more clinical time would increase the amount of learning opportunities for students. However, I don't think that takes into consideration the quality of learning experience. Well-rested medical students will be better able to perform at tasks on-call and retain what they've learned later. Of course shorter shifts don't mean that medical students will never feel stressed or overwhelmed, but decreasing call shifts to 16-hours is an important step to improving students' workload."

Competency/skills based questions

Interviewers ask these types of questions to evaluate whether or not your past experiences have allowed you to develop the capacities they are looking for at the present time. Most commonly, these competencies are stated in individual schools' selection criteria and you should take the time to review this information prior to attending an interview. You should also review your own application to prepare for these types of questions as well. As you go through your experiences, ask yourself what capacities you developed. What did you practice? What did you improve upon? What type of cognitive and non-cognitive skills did this experience require? If you're able to answer these questions while reviewing on your own, you'll find that it is much easier to formulate a persuasive response in an interview.

Example of competency/skills based questions

Tell me about a time when you had to be a leader and a time you had to be a follower?
When did you provide a solution to a challenging problem?
What does professionalism mean to you?
Would other people describe you as a good communicator?
How have you advocated for others in the past?

Sample answer to question four above

I became a resident advisor in my third year of university. At the time, I didn't realize how much advocacy the job required, but I quickly learned how important being assertive, honest, and transparent was to getting the job done well. On a policy level, I had to advocate for dormitory rules with certain residents so that the rights and safety of all the students who lived there was respected. Sometimes that meant having difficult conversations with residents who were breaking rules, but I learned I could be successful applying all policies if I was consistent and fair. On an individual level, I often had to advocate for residents who were in crisis. Many times I became aware of residents who were going through a difficult time and had to seek support on their behalf. It was not an easy job but it emphasized how important it is to be an advocate and gave me a lot of skills to be a successful in the future.

Approach to competency/skills based questions

Generally, you successfully prepare for these types of questions by adequately reflecting on your past experiences. This emphasizes the importance of good preparation. Being able to choose a strong example to highlight the skills the interviewers are looking for is the first step to providing an effective response. Again, it's important to answer the question that is being asked. While you may have several examples of the trait that you are being asked about or the activity you've chosen demonstrates many other competencies, keep your response focused. Make sure to include tangible evidence of how your experience demonstrates the skill in question. For example, in the sample answer provided above, the applicant could have simply said, "I had to advocate for dorm policies and for individual students in crisis." That would have been an incomplete and ineffective answer. A much stronger response is one where you have validated your experience. As well, make sure that you also keep your responses to these types of questions future-oriented. Interviewers are looking for skills that you demonstrated in the past to predict if you will have the competencies necessary to be successful in the future.

Personal type questions

Personal type questions ask you to talk about yourself as an individual. This gives the interviewer an idea of who you are separately from your resume and cover letter. Usually, personal type questions will ask you about your thoughts and actions during a particular time. Because past behavior is often the best predictor of future behavior, your response demonstrates how you will behave as a medical student. There is a tremendous amount of interpersonal interaction in medicine such as, building new relationships with peers and professors, meeting patients, working with members of the healthcare team, engaging with the public, advocating in the public arena, and so on. Even if they seem abstract or superficial, your response to personal type questions demonstrates your problem solving ability, communication style, or how easily you build rapport and work with others.

Example of personal type questions

Tell me about a time when you faced a conflict.
Would you rather work in a group or with a partner?
What are you most proud of and why?
When was the last time you got angry?
Tell me about yourself.

Sample answer to "Tell me about yourself"

I would describe myself as hardworking, thoughtful, and outgoing. I'm the oldest of three boys and was raised by my mom and dad in a mid-sized town. Growing up, my brothers and I played hockey and did karate and I have a lot of happy memories traveling to games and sparring matches together. I wasn't the most athletic of the three of us so I had to learn to set goals and work towards them if I wanted to keep up with my brothers. Eventually, I learned the value of a strong work ethic even without being rewarded or in competition, and I still believe in that today. My parents were a strong influence on all of us and taught us to show respect to everyone we meet and to do your best at everything you do. We're a very close family and one of my favorite things to do is share dinner together because my mom is such a great cook. I don't know if I would have survived undergrad if my mom hadn't taught me to cook and passed on her recipes. It was really difficult to leave home when I started university. But, I really believed that I was going into a program that was going to best prepare me for medicine, and I thought the distance would help me mature. I really enjoyed my undergraduate years. I learned that even though I liked the familiarity and structure of home, it's important to try to venture out my comfort zone to grow. Now I love meeting new people and trying new things.

Approach to personal type questions

Personal type questions ask about universal human experiences. Everyone has faced conflict, has accomplishments, has been angry, and had to work alone or with others. It would reflect poorly on you if you could not come up with a response. One of the most common personal type questions is "Tell me about yourself." This is not only one of the first questions you'll be asked at a panel/traditional interview, but one of the hardest of the interview questions; it is always advisable to prepare a response prior to a panel/traditional or modified panel interview. Many applicants are tempted to rely on details from their resume or cover letter to answer this. Others focus their response heavily on their strengths or suitability. Medical schools can look at your paper application if they want to know these things; they're asking you this question to get to know you as an individual. Resumes don't get admitted to medical school. People get admitted to medical school.

While your experiences and skills should be a part of your response because they are important aspects of who you are, your emphasis should be on giving an overall impression of who you are personally and professionally. Keep your response concise but well rounded. You can organize your response chronologically and discuss your significant life experiences from childhood until the present day. You can also structure your response by saying how you would describe yourself and why.

Choosing what to say in your response can be anxiety provoking. It's challenging to balance being open and engaged without over-sharing; it can be difficult sharing intimate details of one's life, particularly if they were traumatic. Sometimes applicants feel like they don't have anything interesting or worthy to mention about themselves. Interviewers don't have a score sheet when marking these questions. You can share what you feel comfortable sharing as long as you give an idea of what kind of person you are. You can begin preparing your response by including answers to these questions: How would you describe yourself? How would your friends describe you? What are you passionate about? What do you like to do in your spare time? What's important to you? Why did you make some of the decisions you did?

Personal type questions based on your application

These questions allow you to further describe the non-cognitive skills that you gained from the activities you listed on your resume, activities sketch, or personal letter. Typically, interviewers have reviewed your application and will inquire about activities where they seek a more detailed explanation. These questions have many purposes. First, they can verify that your experience actually was enriching and wasn't simply an act of "resume padding." You might be asked what you learned in an experience or specific details about your roles and responsibilities within a certain activity. Second, it can be an opportunity to build even more connections between your life experience and your suitability to the medical profession. For example, you could be asked how a previous research project taught you to appraise and evaluate other research and evidence. Make sure that you reinforce what you've already stated on paper as well as answer the new question being posed. Just as with competency-based questions, it's important to review your application prior to your interview to refresh your memory and anticipate these types of questions.

Example of personal type questions based on your application

I read in your personal letter that you had a challenging time adjusting to your first year of university and this is why your marks are lower compared to the rest of your schooling. Attending medical school will be another big adjustment for you. What makes you think you'll be prepared for the new challenges you'll encounter?

Sample answer

"I can understand why that's an important question because you need to have confidence that I have the capability to perform well academically as a medical student. I know that physicians have to be adaptable and level headed. I also know now how important it is to be aware of my own limitations and be open to seeking help if I need to. Since first year, I have learned time management and organizational skills necessary to meet increased work demands. I've also learned to take good care of myself

so I'm physically able to deal with stress better and I make sure to keep a better balance between my personal and professional life. This has helped me handle similarly stressful situations since my first year of school and has prepared me for the next stage of my career. To answer your question, I've had to reflect on all of my experiences – not just my first year in university – to assess whether or not I was mature and prepared for medical school before I decided to apply and I truly believe I am prepared to deal with new and challenging situations. "

Approach to personal type questions based on your application

These types of questions are asked by assessors who are familiar with your application. It's not helpful to restate what you've already expressed on paper. Essentially, you want to answer the question that has been asked of you by providing new insight into the skills and qualities you developed. Keep your response future oriented. This means that you elaborate on the activity such that you make it clear to an interviewer how your past experience will serve you in medical school. Your response should include statements like, "Because of what I learned (or developed, gained, practiced, and so on), I believe I will be able to…" or "I learned the importance of (a certain skill or quality) and make sure that I practice it every opportunity I can."

Quirky type questions

Hopefully you've noticed that you can prepare for most type of interview questions. Quirky type questions, however, are almost impossible to anticipate. These are the questions that seem to come out of the blue or are completely unrelated to your application or anything that has been previously discussed in the interview. You might be asked to talk about the last book you read, what color best describes your personality, or what you would do with ten-thousand dollars. These questions are intended to gauge how you think on your feet and respond to unexpected situations. It's easy to overthink quirky questions, too. Sometimes, these are used as icebreakers or to relieve any anxiety between you and the interviewer. While it's true that you can't rehearse your answers to quirky type questions, you can certainly prepare for them. Including these types of questions in your preparation will help you control nerves when asked surprising or disarming questions and your practice will give you the experience to think and react quickly.

Examples of quirky type questions

How many unread emails do you have in your inbox?
How do you take your coffee or tea?
If you could be any animal, what would you be and why?
If you could travel anywhere in the world, where would you go?
What is the top item on your bucket list?

Approach to these types of questions

Again, while you might not be able to anticipate what is being asked in quirky questions, you can certainly practice the skills necessary to perform well. Though these are seemingly random questions, they can be asked of anyone in any scenario. Almost everyone has email, has a coffee or tea preference, knows at least a few animals, has thought about traveling, and reflected on things they want to do in life. You will be expected to formulate an answer; unfortunately, "I don't know," doesn't count. Begin by taking a deep, calming breath and allow yourself time to pause. Avoid the urge to answer what you think an assessor wants to hear. For some questions, you might need time to gather your thoughts and that's perfectly reasonable. You can do this by saying, "That's an interesting question. I need a few seconds to get my thoughts in order." You can use the first thing that comes to mind as long as it is appropriate, logical, and you can offer a brief explanation.

Final Thought

Interviews are one of the biggest and most difficult steps in your application process. It's important to prepare early – and prepare wisely. Make sure you set aside enough time to get a broad background in important interview topics and familiarize yourself with the types of questions you could be asked. Practice an organized and thoughtful approach to providing a response. Every applicant will feel nervous on test day. It's normal! If you anticipate feeling anxious and work on managing stress as you prepare, you'll be able to go to your interviews comfortable and confident and leave a great impression on your interviewers.

For additional preparation tips and sample questions visit BeMo's online interview resource guide at MedSchoolInterviewQuestions.com

CHAPTER VIII

Mature and Non-Traditional Students Chapter

The practice of medicine is an art, not a trade; a calling, not a business; a calling in which your heart will be exercised equally with your head.

-*Sir William Osler*

Medicine is a profession that rewards mature, thoughtful, and independent people. While it may be a longer, windier road, to enter medicine from a non-science background or as a mature learner, or both, being a non-traditional applicant and future practitioner positively impacts the medical community and the lives of patients served by such unique doctors.

This chapter will:

- *Help you understand if you fall into the mature/non-traditional learner category*
- *Assist you in identifying what medical schools want in a mature/non-traditional applicant*
- *Identify your weaknesses as an applicant, and*
- *Help you plan to improve your application over time.*

There are two groups of mature and non-traditional learners. The first group is comprised of people who studied in non-science degree programs but always knew they would aim to get into medical school. If you are in this category, you may have slotted in science courses alongside your political science, western civilization, music, or economics courses so that you met the prerequisite courses needed by some schools, and simultaneously prepared for the MCAT. Ideally, you wrote the MCAT in second year and rewrote if needed. If you are in this category you have also volunteered in medicine-related fields and attained extraordinary grades. There is probably also ample evidence on your resume that you are committed to medicine. People with your academic profile are found in every medical school on the continent and contribute significantly to the texture of the class. Your arts and science training allows you to think broadly and systematically and your reliance on first principles to understand, and not just memorize, the material make you a unique candidate. You are, however, likely new to concepts like 'problem-based learning' but can adapt over time.

Who is this chapter for and who is it NOT for?

This chapter is not for this first group of people. This chapter is for people who did not plan to get into medical school until later in life, have a non-science background and/or have special circumstances, which prevented them from taking the well-trodden path to medical school. This chapter will address special circumstances but will not address equity and diversity in medicine because this topic requires its own focus. The chapter is for mature and non-traditional learners who do not qualify for any other equity or diversity admissions program, such as those based on ethnicity, language, and community of origin or ability.

The most essential message of this chapter is that mature and non-traditional learners can get into medical school if they have strong academic assets and market themselves well. Every piece of advice about applying to medical school in this book also applies to mature and non-traditional students. Without strong academic assets, the chances of success plummet but there are ways to improve your GPA and MCAT scores to allow the adult learner's strengths to shine. Medical schools do not have quotas for mature and non-traditional learners applying outside of a specific diversity or equity admissions program. They accept mature and non-traditional learners entirely at their discretion so admission is by no means a foregone conclusion.

Do mature and non-traditional learners get into medical school?

Medical schools across North America accept a wide variety of students as long as they meet all of the admission criteria with some rare exceptions. However, it is true that the vast majority of admitted students to MD programs are in their early 20s and have a science degree. If you don't belong to this group, there still could be a home for you at medical schools around the continent.

For example, in the USA, at Johns Hopkins School of Medicine, 17% had a non-science undergraduate degree. At Case Western Reserve University in Cleveland, 30% had a non-science, non-math undergraduate degree and 15% had a graduate degree. For Canada,18 of the 288 students accepted to the University of British Columbia's medical school were non-science, non-engineering, and non-public health. At McMaster, 26 students of the 206 accepted students had non-traditional academic backgrounds. These numbers vary year to year, but you can be assured that medical schools are hunting for non-traditional students that can adapt and thrive in medical training. The kind of degree is less important than the grades earned.

At Johns Hopkins, the oldest member of the class was 35 and the average age was 23. The eldest member of the class at Boston University School of Medicine was 34 but a member of a previous class was 40 years old on admission. At the University of British Columbia, 44 percent of the entering class was over 24. At McMaster University, approximately nine percent of the class was over 26 years old. Dalhousie University's class has an MD candidate that is 39 years old and the average age on admission for that Class was 24. There are a handful of MD students in their 40s and 50s admitted annually to one or more medical schools around the continent but these admissions are rare. After the age of 50, it can become difficult for a public medical school to justify the expense of training versus the potential for public good given that a new medical learner could spend 10 years learning before they are able to really give back to a system.

What is the most important thing mature and non-traditional learners must do when applying to medical school?

If you are a mature or non-traditional learner, you have one top job when applying to medical school. You must be able to answer this question: **Why do you want to be a doctor?** You must answer with conviction, purpose and detail. This is the most important question for two reasons. First and foremost, knowing why you want to be a doctor is in itself a source of motivation. On those tough days where you are wading through new topics in an MCAT prep course and everyone else is way ahead of you, you need to know why you are putting yourself through the effort. It is worth it, but only if you know why you want to be a doctor.

Mature and non-traditional learners have to prove that they can handle the work. If you have a 2.9 GPA taken in part-time courses and middling MCAT scores, it is hard for a medical school to assess your scholarly competencies. Everyone knows that GPA doesn't fully capture intellect, but it does capture intellect, discipline and some contextual factors in sum. In the coming sections, we will review an approach to medical school admissions for people with various academic trajectories and records.

The second reason you must know why you want to be a doctor is so that you can target your volunteer and extracurricular efforts to fit with your story in a cohesive, sensical way. Your resume may have nothing that indicates a desire to work with people, an interest in physiology or pharmacology or even experience with hands-on skills, so you should get yourself involved in activities that allow you to expand upon these categories.

You should spend time finding volunteer and research opportunities that demonstrate empathy, critical thinking, ability to learn in a clinical setting, and professionalism.

Review the Essential Skills and Abilities Required for the Study of Medicine to support your efforts. You should not, however, focus all of your energy on trying to be like the traditional students in every way. Your story matters when admissions committees are trying to figure out if you fit at their school. Highlight that your story is unique but buttress it with authentic efforts to demonstrate your commitment to the field.

He who studies medicine without books sails
an uncharted sea, but he who studies medicine
without patients does not go to sea at all.
- WILLIAM OSLER

Mature and non-traditional learners tend to have had more comprehensive experiences interfacing with the rest of humanity. They may have experienced less privilege than an average medical student, traveled more and experienced more. They may find it easier to situate their interest in medicine inside the human experience. This is where doctors and patients meet and medical schools, increasingly, understand that students who 'get' people make excellent doctors.

Which kinds of mature and non-traditional learners do medical schools want?

Medical schools describe the types of students they want to apply to their programs using very particular language. Mature learners often see themselves in those descriptions and believe their chances of admission are very good as a result. However, most medical schools consider these personal aptitudes and characteristics as supplementary to the high GPA and MCAT scores and not more important than these academic achievements. That is, a mature learner without a high GPA or MCAT score has to be extraordinary. Each medical school publishes descriptors for mature/non-traditional applicants that the school is trying to attract. We encourage you to look at the specific description of the school you're interested in. Through reviewing a number of these descriptors, certain themes arise that are universally applicable:

Theme 1: Healing and service

Maybe you're a mature student who is starving for an opportunity to help people solve problems and live better lives. Medicine could be a perfect match for you. Ask yourself how your life has set you up for this opportunity. Identify which aspects of your personality and which of your strengths will allow you to excel in a service profession. Spend time writing about the importance of healing and service in your own life's purpose so that when you write your application, the medical schools see you as being compatible with their avatar.

Theme 2: Professionalism

In Sandeep Jauhar's perspective piece in the New England Journal of Medicine on mature and non-traditional learners, he shares the opinion of one of his older classmates around professionalism and older students. He states, "for most interns, this is the first job they've ever had...They have no concept of being a professional. When you're an older student, you have a different perspective. You spend less time whining that the world is unfair." If you are a mature student, your strengths lie in experiential learning, possibly even self-directed graduate studies, and knowing what it's like to have a career. This makes you much more like your everyday patient than many other applicants. Professionalism is, first and foremost, about competency. The only standardized way to assess competency of a medical school applicant is to use academic metrics like the GPA or MCAT. However, professionalism is also, according to the College of Physicians and Surgeons, about "codes of ethics and a commitment to clinical competence, the embracing of appropriate attitudes and behaviors, integrity, altruism, personal well-being, and the promotion of the public good." Mature students have had more time to have more adult experiences with ethics and professionalism. Non-traditional students are capable of seeing these issues from many angles.

Theme 3: Well-Rounded / Life Experience

Mature students should know that the algorithms to determine admissions don't technically capture "life experience" in an obvious way but medical schools almost all say that they want well-rounded learners. This can feel like a mixed message to an applicant but it is because universities want to retain a level of discretion when assessing non-academic requirements. You need to focus on channeling your experience into stellar personal statements, CASPer writing (if you are applying to schools using this admissions tool) and, if you are invited, interview skills that illustrate your experience and adaptability. Your experience should also segue naturally into an explanation of why you want to be a doctor, with specific mention of why medical experiences are the right ones for your life.

How do mature and non-traditional learners do in medical school and in medicine?

Non-traditional learners - those with non-science backgrounds - are typically at par with their science-trained colleagues at graduation from the MD programs. This is why most medical schools continue to accept these students. However, the question of maturity is different. Medical schools have almost always accepted a small number of mature applicants annually and, on balance, find that they enhance the student body and have better bedside manner, but come with their own challenges.

A study from the United Kingdom by Oyne and Ben-Shiomo found that doctors who graduated from medical school older than 29 years had greater difficulty advancing through their specialist training programs. The study looked at performance records for over 38 000 graduates. The authors proposed a number of explanations for their findings:

1. *Older trainees have more commitments outside of work.*
2. *Older trainees may choose a specialty in order to make their training compatible with the work of their spouse.*
3. *Older trainees may perform less well on certification exams.*
4. *Older trainees may have less social support compared to the camaraderie enjoyed by the younger trainees.*

5. *Older trainees may be more confident leaving their specialty training program because they've made previous career changes and find the transitions more tolerable than would a more junior doctor.*

Jauhar proposes (http://www.nejm.org/doi/full/10.1056/NEJMp 0802264), however, that older medical learners may have less energy and drive to learn in spite of the regular distractions of life. He also posits that older learners are less apt to conform to hospital pecking orders and find themselves in trouble with the school's administration. He quotes Lawrence Smith, former dean of New York's Mount Sinai, "[Mature learners] are more self-confident...They're more conscious of what they want to do with their time. They're less willing to just suck it up and go through the rote aspects of medical training. They are the ones you see in the dean's office saying, 'Don't inflict this horrible teacher on me.'"

What should I do to get into medical school?

Getting into medical school as a mature or non-traditional learner can be a murky, uncertain process. Many people give up. In this section, we will review plans for gaining acceptance based on a few common mature/non-traditional applicant profiles.

All mature applicants should explain their 'special circumstances' in their personal statements. See the Chapter on Application Components to review how to approach these explanations. Always be sure to return to the themes of service and healing, professionalism and lived experience when explaining any circumstances, as these cohere with the desired applicant descriptions for the vast majority of schools.

When you are putting together your plan for applications, it is important that you're narrowing down your school pool to only those for which you meet admission criteria, or will soon meet admission criteria.

It is very important that mature learners approach medical training with a gracious, open mind towards their younger colleagues and foster in themselves a disciplined, thoughtful approach to studying which reflects the principles of adult learning: internal motivation, experiential learning, goal-oriented, relevancy-oriented, practical and desire for respect.

Conclusion

If you are a mature or non-traditional learner, it is possible to get into medical school. But, getting in is going to be more difficult than for a traditional applicant. You cannot just submit an application and hope for the best. Spending significant time thinking through your narrative, planning ways to strengthen your CV, and understanding more about what makes an ideal doctor is important. Figure out why you want to be a doctor and allow this to serve as your mission statement as you plan your approach. Take the time - years if needed - to meet as many eligibility criteria as possible. Expect rejection. Leave your ego at the door and continue to apply anyway. Even if you came from a high-ranking career in another discipline, you probably need support in planning your application. Time and effort up front can help you avoid the classic mistakes of mature and non-traditional students and improve your chances of acceptance. To learn more how BeMo can help you make your application stand out visit BeMoAcademicConsulting.com.

CHAPTER IX

Case Studies: Do as they say AND as they do.

This chapter will provide you with several case studies of past successful medical school applicants who have now gone on to study medicine or are currently practicing as physicians. Although everyone's journey to medical school is unique and distinct, there are some overlapping key elements that will become apparent after you review the various cases. As you read these cases, try to remind yourself of the concepts and ideas that were discussed in earlier parts of the book and attempt to appreciate how each successful candidate incorporated the concepts in their plan and road map to medical school. We hope that the stories shared here will inspire you to continue on your path to becoming the "good doctor" that is so desperately needed in our society.

One important note before we begin, as you read this section, you will notice that the majority of the MCAT scores are based on the old MCAT scale/scoring system. This is no surprise as the new MCAT was only instituted in 2015. For comparison's sake, we have included the rough score equivalents to the new MCAT as well as percentiles in brackets after the original scores. Please note, the AAMC firmly states that these conversions are not entirely accurate. The conversions are offered only as a reference and convenience for you.

Case One: Dr. Helena Frischtak, B.Sc., M.D.
Bachelor of Science (Wisconsin-Madison)

Like many others, there wasn't a distinct moment when I realized I wanted to be a doctor, but right from my first year of college, in the United States, I followed the pre-med track. I had grown up in Rio de Janeiro, and even though I attended an international school, college in the U.S. was a huge change. Not making my situation any easier was the fact I wound up at a gigantic undergrad institution: the University of Wisconsin-Madison.

UW-Madison was an amazing place, overflowing with resources and opportunities. But it lacked good advising and mentorship to make students *aware* of these opportunities. I didn't realize at the time, but I was completely lost. Thus, I took longer than most to get on the strategic boat of a pre-med student. I only started volunteering my junior year, when I discovered the Madison House, an organization that many American universities have to compile all volunteer opportunities for students. I only started shadowing physicians my summer after junior year. And, even though I found a research project early on, my time in that neuroscience lab had been directionless: I didn't realize I should aim to have results for a poster or oral presentation.... I just went through the motions of the experiments.

Not surprisingly, when it came time to apply to medical school as a junior in college, I didn't feel ready. I had taken an MCAT prep course but hadn't found it useful. When I opened the AMCAS application, I didn't know what to write about. So I decided to take time off after university before applying. I felt it was better to wait and get it right than put myself out there sloppily.

As college graduation loomed in the horizon, I was sure of one thing only: I wanted to move to New York City, where several of my high school friends were. To my parents' despair, I arrived in NYC without a job or a plan. But as they tend to do, things worked out. My father worked with a Portuguese economist back in Brazil, whose sister was a neuroscientist at a cancer hospital in town. It took several months, but she referred me for a position as a research assistant at Memorial Sloan-Kettering Cancer Hospital. During that year, I also accrued experiences for my CV: more shadowing, more volunteering, etc. By the following summer, I felt ripe to apply to medical school. That would mean a total of two gap years by the time I enrolled as a medical student.

I didn't have impressive MCAT scores nor a stellar GPA. But I had a unique application. I had always been an analytical person, and had spent a lot of time thinking about the patient encounters and hospital systems I had witnessed, both in the US and in Brazil. Thus, I had a lot of insight to share in my personal statement and secondary applications. Multiple doctors remarked on the maturity my writing displayed. I still felt tremendously insecure, due to not having high numbers. The entire time I worked on my application, there was a voice inside me saying I may never get to be a doctor. If you feel insecure too, know you are not alone.

I applied to 25 medical schools and received 7 interview invitations. I cried when I saw that first email with an interview invitation. The application process may feel esoteric at times - we send all this information out to the world and are not entirely sure who, if anyone, is reading our words. So when interview invitations appear in our email box, it is quite re-assuring. I attended 6 interviews and was accepted to 4 medical schools. Even though my dream school rejected me, multiple acceptances felt like the biggest success I could fathom. I was elated, and my parents – after that initial disgruntlement about my NYC move – were beaming with pride.

In med school, you are surrounded by intelligent, ambitious, and caring people. You may not get along with everybody, but you realize most people around you are good-hearted. I made great friends, and I bet you will too. The shear experience of going through such life-forming years together brings you very close.

However, the material is hard, and it's a LOT at once - we have to train our brain to memorize dozens of lectures in little time, and organize this material such that we recall it in exams. I remember several evenings, arriving home after spending 10-12 hours at the library and just crying. I didn't even know why I cried - it was some cathartic experience, relieving the stress from that day. But each year in med school is different than the year prior, and you feel progressively more confident. It's not an easy journey, but it's an incredibly fulfilling one. I have graduated med school and still feel nostalgic for most of it - including the countless hours studying as a first-year.

Residency application is not as stressful - because unlike when you apply to med school, you *know* you will likely get into *a* residency, even if not your dream program. I decided to take a year off to do research while in med school, through a fellowship called Doris Duke. I lived in Peru during that time and it was an unforgettable experience. After med school graduation, I took another year off and came to New Zealand, where I currently write this. This second move was personal - I came to accompany my partner Dan, who had to be here for professional reasons. In NZ, I pursued both clinical and research experiences. I will be submitting my residency application in two months to return to the US next year. That means that when I finally start residency, my peers will be people who were two years below me in med school! However, I don't see myself as getting behind. On the contrary, both my year in Peru and my year in NZ have added tremendously to me - and for me, it's about the journey, not the end point.

Case Two: Dr. Izu Ibe, MD (Orthopedic Surgery)
GPA: 3.4
MCAT: high 20s (503-509)

My road to medical school, like many, was relatively tortuous and convoluted. My planning did not begin till my Junior year in College when I realized that being a doctor was the career for me. This did not become evident until I shadowed a physician whose office was near my school. At that point, I had to face reality, I had no research or volunteer experience, and I had just figured out that there was an exam named the MCAT. I decided to not rush and take the MCAT at the end of my senior year and take a year off (now known as the gap year) while I applied to medical school. This was after I graduated and spending time relearning many things seemed like an arduous task. I initially took a prep course, but this did not work for me. After I took the MCAT the first time and did not like my score I embarked on a mission to take it again. This time I did as many review questions as I could and tried to always study intensely as opposed to passively going over things. This increased my weakest portion by about 4 points allowing me to comfortably apply. Sometimes if you take the MCAT multiple times some programs will take your highest point score in the sections and total it.

In my gap year, while preparing for the MCAT, I considered a couple of things, teaching at a high school or going to school for another program. I ended up deciding on the latter. After taking my MCAT the second time, I applied to medical schools as well as a program in cytotechnology. Either choice would have been good and would have left me with a lot to speak about in my application and during interviews, but the program was essentially a post-bac, and it provided me with medical school-type courses, and doing well in them allowed me to tell medical schools that I could tolerate their demanding curriculum. Another reason this was a good choice is because my grade point average was not superb coming out of college, but once you do a post-bac program, admissions committees, at times, overlook your college GPA and pay more attention to your post-bac GPA; the caveat with that is that you have to do well.

In College I participated in division 1 athletics. This made it difficult to do many other activities but I was able to fit in some things in the summers and whenever I had free time. I shadowed a physician, as mentioned previously, who worked close to my University. I went to his office once or twice a month for a period of six months. During this time, I also participated in a summer research program that gave me some research experience and introduced me to the scientific process. I signed up to volunteer at a nearby hospital and went once a month for a full year. I believe shadowing and volunteering in medical settings are important activities to partake in when applying for medical school. They both show that you have a vested interest in helping people and learning about the field of medicine. Research is not mandatory but it never hurts to have participated in a project or two.

Being a doctor has been something I have always wanted. It took me till my Junior year in college to realize that and make a final decision. Deciding late, knowing I was behind many of my colleagues who had essentially built a resume from their first day of undergraduate studies was one of my motivators. Another motivating factor was meeting my guidance counselor who told me that I would not make it to medical school because I did not have a 4.0 grade point average. She was wrong! As it turns out, medical schools look at applicants holistically and as a total package, not just as numbers on a paper. Obviously, the higher the grade point average the better, but you can make it to medical school if your GPA is not perfect. Many individuals have circumstances that come up during undergraduate studies, some people work multiple jobs, take care of family members, or have that one bad grade in freshman year that weighs them down. This is natural and understandable.

As a high school student, I enjoyed studying biological sciences. I never really had as much a liking for other things, but I always had a passion for the sciences and that trend continued when I began College. It seemed natural for me. It is important to note that, you do not have to be a biology major to apply or get into medical school. As a matter of fact, many programs want a mixed class with varying experiences so alternative majors might work in your favor. The traditional pre-med pathway is important, sure, but sometimes the courses are significantly harder and taking a tougher course might back fire because even though you may be at the top of your class for a course with a 'B', when the admissions committees see it, they only see a 'B.'

How did I maximize my academic performance as an undergraduate? This is a tough one to advise on. Everyone learns and absorbs materials differently. I think the important thing to focus on is how to identify what kind of learner you are. Do you like pictures, videos, writings... Do you prefer to highlight, make flash cards, or just make tables? Take the time in college when it is less strenuous to identify these things as it will make the transition to medical school much smoother for you.

All and all, at the time of application my GPA from my university was a 3.24, and a 4.0 for the post-bac program I was enrolled in during my gap year. My overall science GPA was a 3.4 and my MCAT score was in the high 20s (503-509, 61-79rd percentile,). When it came to actually completing applications I decided to approach it very patiently as it was a very difficult and stressful process. Once you submit, you are left pondering "will they contact you? Will they not? Will they invite you for an interview?" This can also be a tad stressful, but it is best to simply enjoy the process and wait for responses. There is no point in stressing!

When you do get an opportunity, be sure to pounce and schedule interviews as soon as you can. Do not be shy to communicate with programs directly, especially those that you are most interested in. Let them know that you really like them after your interview by sending a thank you letter, etc. When it came to preparing for interviews, I preferred to not practice for them in the traditional manner. I usually like things to come out freely and unrehearsed, and I can afford to take this approach because I think quick on my feet and I rarely get flustered in tough situations. This is not the same for everyone and if you feel that you are someone who needs the practice then you need to have a sit down and practice answering interview style questions, especially MMI types. Instead of formally practicing, I thought about and documented my strengths and weaknesses and thought about ways to incorporate them into answers or questions that I might be asked. But again, take the time to prepare, whichever way suites you best.

In the end I found myself at NYMC and after 4 grueling years, I am now an orthopedics resident at Yale. Although the path I took was a bit unconventional, the end result was exactly what I wanted.

Case Three: Dr. Natalie Lidster, RN, MD (Anesthesiology)
Bachelor of Science in Nursing (Thompson Rivers)
GPA: 3.8
MCAT: Physical 10 (127), CARS 12 (129), Biological 11 (128).

I'm writing this after graduating from medical school and at the start of my first year of residency, but I still can't believe I'm here! I took a roundabout road and had a few bumps along the way but that hasn't changed how unbelievably lucky I feel to be a doctor.

Growing up, I did well in elementary and high school and was involved in a lot of activities. I was lucky to have had lots of resources at school and positive direction from my friends and family. Looking back, I didn't have to think too hard about the future: there was always another grade, another field hockey season, or another annual school play. Maybe that's why, when the time came to choose what to study in university, I felt like the rug was pulled out from underneath me. This was something I would have to figure out on my own. My friends were getting excited to study all over the country and I wasn't even sure if I wanted to go to university right out of high school. My full schedule now looked empty and it was daunting thinking of how I was going to fill it.

I ended up enrolling in a general science program at Thompson Rivers University (TRU), a smaller school in my hometown because it seemed like the right choice. I liked my high school science courses. I could save a lot of money living at home. I wouldn't have to make any big adjustments to moving to a new city. I was completely overwhelmed. The courses were far more challenging than I was used to, professors seemed far more distant than my high school teachers, and it was intimidating to make new friends and try new activities. I finished my first semester disappointed in myself.

I talked about this with my parents and they were extremely supportive. I knew they were hesitant to give advice because I was at an age where it was important to begin solving problems and making decisions independently. But I was still hoping to have things figured out for me, although that was impossible. Still, I did learn a few things. Yes, I did have to do homework even if no one was checking it. Yes, there were ways to get help in courses if I needed. Yes, I had to put myself out there if I wanted to make a new network of friends and activities but it was worth it. We also talked about the importance of goal setting and prioritizing. They encouraged me to reflect on what I felt I was good at and what I felt good doing and decide on a course of study and career path after that.

One of my good friends at the time was in the nursing program. I liked hearing her stories about school and she seemed so happy to be doing her work. I was proud of her and I wanted that feeling for myself. I was able to enter into the nursing program in my second year of university. Like my friend, I found it rewarding feeling like I could help others and I enjoyed learning about anatomy and physiology, pharmacology, as well as structure and delivery of healthcare. By that time, I had made the adjustment to my new academic pressures and was performing well. Still, there were aspects of school that didn't feel like a good fit. Some of this was because I needed to mature and develop as a professional, but I began to question whether I was in the right field. I wanted to have a deeper understanding of the science behind the decisions that get made in healthcare and different skills to carry them out. I thought the challenge of diagnosing and prescribing treatments was stimulating and I wanted to take on that responsibility. Sometimes I worried that leaving nursing would be misinterpreted as having a negative opinion of that profession or that medicine offered me "more". But being a nurse is providing care and healing to people in need; it is a true human service performed by talented, hardworking professionals. I was and still am so lucky to have nurses as my colleagues, truly, but I wanted to provide that same level of care in a different job. Someone once told me about the concept of the therapeutic use of self. It's a way of helping others by using the best parts of yourself, including your knowledge and skills as well as your personality. That really resonated with me. Some people find that in nursing and I found that in medicine.

I decided to finish my nursing degree but I returned to TRU a few months later to complete pre-requisite courses and apply to medical school. The decision to pursue a career in medicine can be a stressful one. It's very competitive and that can be difficult. I was lucky that it gave me a motivation that I didn't have before. I was very passive in high school and lost when I began university, but I became focused and determined. I had learned that failing to prioritize and plan caused me to make decisions that weren't right for me and I wanted to do things differently this time around. My grades would be my weakest area so I committed to increasing my GPA: I invested in a tutor for my more challenging courses, and selected electives based on what I was most interested in so that I had more enthusiasm for studying. I wanted to demonstrate that I had academic potential through my extracurricular activities so I volunteered as a tutor and helped a former professor with a research project. After I completed my pre-requisites, I prepared for the MCAT by taking a preparation course online and supplemented my knowledge using Khan Academy videos on YouTube. I also made sure to do lots of timed practice exams. I was so relieved when that hurdle was behind me!

And then it came time to apply. My GPA was 3.8 although my average in pre-requisite courses was less because I had taken a few in my disastrous first year. I scored an 10 (127-128, 79th percentile) in physical sciences, 12 (129-130, 98-99th percentile,) in CARS, 11 (128-129, 88th percentile,) in biological sciences and an S in the written portion as they still included that at the time. I was most proud of my extracurricular activities. I had experience in different areas: work experience, research, volunteering, athletics, and arts. One of the things that probably stood out was my experience of performance and drama. Since childhood, I took drama lessons and performed in a local arts festival and school plays. As I got older, I completed formal exams in theatre and performance. In university, I began instructing students of my own and volunteering at an elementary school with kids who had an interest in drama. I believe my application demonstrated that I was dedicated and committed to something and was successful in it. Furthermore, I had shared that enthusiasm in areas where I also showed leadership and community service. I think that made schools think that I would have the same success if I had the same enthusiasm for medicine.

I so desperately wanted to get in and I thought I would maximize my chances by applying to every school in Canada. I found it tedious looking at each individual school's website for their particular eligibility requirements, admission statistics, and application procedures. It was worth it to know which schools were realistic options for me and to tailor my application to their selection criteria. One of the challenges I faced completing applications was questioning whether I was using the right terminology for my activity sketch or if I was categorizing activities correctly. I received some good advice at the time, which was to focus more on my description of activities and, once I started to emphasize what I learned from each activity, the process started to feel easier.

I received interviews to the University of British Columbia (UBC), for which I was considered in-province, and McMaster University. With two opportunities, I wanted to make the most of my chances. To prepare, I read "Doing Right" and practiced with other applicants. My parents simulated timed interviews for me. Both of them are counselors and spend a lot of time in professional development so I trusted their opinion. As well, I listened to a lot of podcasts about medical ethics, issues in healthcare, and current events. I had to drive a lot for my work so this was an easier way of brushing up on important topics than reading. Finally, at the end of the application process, I received offers of admission to both UBC and McMaster. I was ecstatic. I was going to do what I thought I would be good at and what I felt good doing. I loved both schools and had a hard time choosing between the two. After a lot of reflection, I decided to attend McMaster so that I could graduate in three years. Attending school in Hamilton, Ontario also gave me an opportunity to be more independent after living at home all my life. The decision worked out well for me. I'm still as ecstatic as the day I found out I got in.

I hope future applicants know how important it is to know who they are. I would like to pass on the advice from my parents: **know what you're good at and what feels good to do.** This will help you decide the best course of study, what activities and experiences to pursue, and what schools are the best choices for you. As a prospective student, you'll have to take a hard look at your application and realistically evaluate your likelihood of admission. It was tough for me to know that there were blights on my transcript and that there were schools for which I didn't have much of a chance to be admitted. However, identifying these weaknesses helped me to address them and create a stronger application. Remember that knowing who you are as an applicant is different from knowing who you are as a person. If you feel confident in who you are as a person and your ability to do well in medicine, you'll have the ability to withstand the pressures and challenges you'll face as an applicant. More significantly, you'll have the clarity to find your passion, the enthusiasm to apply this passion to medicine, and successfully make it to medical school and beyond.

Case Four: Dr. Lauren Prufer B.Sc., MD

Bachelor of Science (Queen's)
Doctor of Medicine (Western)

There are a wide variety of paths into medicine, and everyone's journey is slightly different. My own application story is no exception, but I hope that by sharing it with you, I will be able to pass on some valuable lessons I learned along the way and improve your chances of becoming an excellent candidate.

My journey through medicine is difficult for me to put into words: it has been both mind-numbingly typical and infinitely unique. I wanted to be a doctor from a very young age and, though I did consider other careers along the way, I ended up doing a pre-medical-type degree at Queen's University in Canada on the picturesque shores of Lake Ontario. I had been debating between science and engineering, but science had won out by a hair and so there I was. To be honest, I was mostly just over-the-moon excited to be going to my first choice school and was already too busy plotting my varsity rugby debut to be overly worried about my choice of major.

For the most part, my first year went very well. I met some of my best friends, made the varsity rugby squad and even had pretty good grades. My second year, however, was a lot more difficult. With a lab or assignment due almost every day of the week, the course load increased precipitously. Between my two-a-day rugby practices and issues back home, I struggled to keep afloat. In order to keep up, I cut back on sleep and studied during every waking moment. I started spending all of my time in the library, becoming more and more miserable. By the end of the year, I had decided that if this was what I had to do to get into medicine, it probably wasn't worth it. I vowed that my third year would be different.

I still wrote my MCAT that summer as planned, but returned to school in the fall on a mission to re-structure my life and have a better year. I backed out of the hyper-competitive pre-medical degree stream and instead took a more general program, committing to only 2-3 notoriously difficult courses per semester. I filled the rest of my courses with things that were interesting, but also known GPA boosters. I took an even bigger step, and quit rugby. The relationships on the team had started to gnaw at me, and after 6 years of playing, I felt that it was time. To replace the hole in my schedule, I went to clubs night on campus and joined every club that caught my fancy. One of these was varsity cross country, and I haven't stopped running since. I also started volunteering with a variety of organizations, most of them involving teaching or playing with children. Though I wasn't enjoying a lot of my course work, I did enjoy teaching science to others, so it was something that felt right for me to be doing. I slept 8 hours a night. I ate 3 meals a day. I went to studying workshops and learned to be more efficient. I went out on weekends. I stopped going to the library. My grades went back up and I started to enjoy university again.

A little later my MCAT scores came back; I had done well! I celebrated with my housemates and sister in our "ghetto" living room. The "what-if" of medicine started to creep back. I decided to give it a try, but only if I could get in doing the activities I enjoyed. I figured that if I couldn't, then it probably wasn't something I was meant to be doing anyway. So I applied, got three interviews and was wait-listed twice. Soon after, I was accepted at Schulich School of Medicine and Dentistry at the Western University, Canada.

Though I can't guarantee that what worked for me will work for you, I did learn a lot from my time at Queen's and my own medical school application, as well as those of my partner and some of my close friends. I can say that like me, many of the students who I have worked with have had a bad year, or struggled with issues at home while they were away at school. Though I hope my story reassures those of you who have faced similar challenges that a year of bad grades will not ruin your chances of acceptance, I also hope for you to be able to learn from my mistakes, by seeking help as soon as you recognize that you are starting to falter. The other piece of advice that I would like to give you is to above all do what you love. Go to the school you want to go to, take the major you're most interested in and fill your life with things that you are passionate about. Doing the appropriate prerequisites, having good grades and acing your MCAT are all necessary, but otherwise, spend your time pursuing your passions and making the world a better place. For me, that was running competitively and my volunteering. If you pursue the things you love, you will learn more, be more dedicated and, most importantly, mold yourself into a better person and thus, a better candidate.

Case Five: Dr. Ashley White, MD (Family Medicine)
Bachelor of Arts and Science (McMaster)
Master of Public Health (Simon Fraser)
GPA: 3.8
MCAT: Physical 2 (118), CARS 14 (131), Biological 2 (118).

My name is Ashley White and I was a member of the Class of 2015 at McMaster University. I am a family medicine resident at McMaster University in the rural stream at the time of writing this, which means that my training is geared towards the demands of 'rural generalism.' This is the technical term for physicians that have a broad base of technical, managerial and procedural skills that are best suited to providing comprehensive primary care in remote and rural settings.

I chose rural family medicine because I am, myself, from the country. I came from a small town in central Ontario. My high school had almost no academic electives. I had never heard of the IB program (International Baccalaureate, for my rural countrymen). My parents are not university graduates and there are no doctors or lawyers or engineers in my family.

The act of going to university was considered a real accomplishment. So there was no pressure to become a doctor, lawyer or anything else. I only had the self-derived pressure to live fully as an undergraduate. I studied in the Arts & Science Program at McMaster University. This degree is a known entity to some universities in Ontario, but not outside. It is one of the best liberal arts and critical thinking training grounds in Canada and I was fortunate to be accepted in 2003. I held my own academically and I finished with a 3.8 GPA over four years, with a Minor Concentration in Economics.

My most significant error as an undergraduate student was picking extra curricular activities over academics in second year. The competitive rowing season ran from April to November and then we trained a lot over the winter. My first year on the team was also my first time taking physics in university. My program mandated a full year of physics. Our classes were from 8:30am to 10:30am three times per week. So, I would bike down to practice at 5:00am, train from 5:30am to 7:45am, bike home, shower, eat and go to class with two large mugs of coffee. And I fell asleep every single time. On weekends, I worked hard AND played hard but never caught up on sleep. By the end of the year, I was pulling a C+ in a full year of physics, which devastated my GPA. This C+ was the reason I lost McMaster's nomination to the Rhodes Scholarship in my fourth year. The selection committee told me exactly this. That C+ also, in my view, put it in my head that maybe I wasn't very good at science, even though I had done well in calculus and biology in first year. This C+ represented a poor, yearlong decision to value everything else over my grades. It also reflected sheer exhaustion because - as I now know - I am not bad at science.

Through happenstance, trial and error and sheer will, I did a number of things really well when it came to academics:

- **I listened to feedback, particularly on my writing:** The bread and butter of the Arts & Science Program is writing. We wrote all possible forms of prose in every subject, including physics. I was a clean slate stylistically so I just absorbed all criticism about my work. This helped me get better. If I can advise one thing to new undergraduates, it is to move your ego aside and listen to your professors and upper year peers.
- **I went to office hours:** If there was a calculus problem that I could not figure out, I did not ask my peers for the answer. I would sometimes ask them to explain their thinking but this rarely worked for me. I wanted to work through the problems – not just the answers, but also the process – with a tutor. The university hires these people to help you so do take advantage.
- **I gave up on lectures:** I went to university for the first time when laptops weighed one million pounds and the first smartphone was being circulated in Palo Alto, California, not in Hamilton. Even without these distractions, my brain does not process didactic auditory input very well. I have never done well in lectures and by the end of my second year, I stopped going to all non-mandatory

lectures. The point is that everyone has to figure out how their own brain works. There were a few very special professors by whom I was riveted. They used narrative to explain abstract concepts and this was very effective for me. But these professors are few and far between. During lecture time, I would be in the library with a textbook teaching myself the material through practice questions. I needed to get myself straight on the foundational principles and then practice applying them to problem solving. When I did show up to lectures, I was right there with the class. This is, of course, with the exception of the dreaded physics, through which I slept for an entire year. If you like lectures, go to lectures. Don't do what I did just because I got into medical school. Try the approach if you like but do what gets *you* results.

- **I did damage control on group work:** Group work was the bane of my existence as an undergraduate. This is true for most ambitious people who work quickly. Any group work outside of the Arts & Science Program required intensive management. The reality is that every group will have one or two people with high standards who will write a very strong lab report or research essay. The group will have a few slackers who will go completely AWOL for the meetings and not fulfill their commitment. The group will have one or two people who will try really hard but their work will have to be redone. And the group will have one or two capable people who are totally overwhelmed by requirements from other courses. This is how it is. There is no sense in complaining to the professor because they don't care. It has happened every year for them for 20 or more years. Your only hope is damage control. Offer to do a large part of the most technical work. Get it done early and then see who is dropping balls. Offer to pick up their load. Be kind and respectful but everyone will know what is going on. Try your best to work with the people who are capable but overwhelmed and trying but can't keep up. This is where you develop leadership skills and the ability to bring out the best in people. Identify their strengths and empower them to perform very well on a manageable task while you keep the big picture in mind. Do not complain about others' performance because it is rude and ineffective. For the slackers, they may have all sorts of other terrible things going on in their lives. Or they may be lazy. Either way, in your final year of study, you will find out that one or more notorious slackers from your groups got into medical school, law school or some other prestigious professional school. He or she is probably a genius with a lot of support at home and in life. This is life. Move forward.

- **I never asked for a grade to be revised:** There is so much grade inflation at the post-secondary level. It renders all of our grades meaningless. Not everyone deserves an A at everything. It is not your right. If you underperform on an assignment, and you believe the professor does not have a vendetta against you, then accept the grade and do better next time. Do not complain about it. It is entirely reasonable to send an email and ask how you could do better next time. This demonstrates character and clear-sightedness. Do not, under any circumstances, have your parents contact the professor or teaching assistant. This does happen. It happened to me when I was a teaching assistant. It is ridiculous to expect your parents to advocate on your behalf as a university student. This professor will never write you a strong or supportive letter of reference. This professor will dread having you in their senior courses. You will not learn anything from your mistakes and you will not grow. You are in charge of the standards to which you will be held.

I approached my undergraduate degree like a child let loose in a candy store without supervision. I was on the varsity rowing team for two and a half seasons, competing for McMaster at the Canadian university championships. And I was a volunteer with the Emergency First Response Team for four years. I ran the student government elections for one year, which was all consuming and insane. I spent several months of my last two years in Northeast India trying to develop a model of political participation for rural women. This was my most significant research experience and it was a self-directed thesis. To make money, I worked at a shawarma place, taught swimming at a summer camp, worked as a research assistant for three years, including summers, and was a teaching assistant for an Arts & Science course in my fourth year. I did not plan for medical school. Nor did I plan for anything that I could do after I completed my degree. I had no idea what I wanted to do when I finished undergraduate studies. I didn't know why I wanted to be a doctor, a lawyer or anything else.

I took a disorganized approach to planning my academics. I was used to just picking courses that sounded interesting, regardless of my course load or my GPA. I saw everyone else play this strategy game with their courses and I never understood why. So my course selection was that of someone who was directionless, even though I performed well. I never met with an academic counselor. I never sat down and thought, "Hey girl, where are you going with all of this?" I just assumed that I would work hard and figure it out because, until then, that was absolutely my life motto. I had no vision. My theory was that if I worked all out, with 100% energy, at anything that I enjoyed, my life would unfold in a good way. Ten years later, I can see that this is probably a half true.

When fourth year rolled around, I applied to law school at McGill, medicine at McMaster and NOSM, graduate school in economics at McMaster and in public health at Simon Fraser University. Because I saved up no money or time to write the LSAT, MCAT or GRE, I just applied where I met the eligibility criteria. McMaster said no and did not grant an interview. McGill waitlisted me for law school and NOSM waitlisted me for medical school.

But I got into both graduate programs. I felt basically fine about the whole thing because I still had no idea what I wanted to do with my life. And I was really excited about moving to Vancouver. I still consider it a rite of passage for Canadian youth.

I know people who applied to medical school seven or eight times. I know them because they were my preceptors when I myself went through medical school. They were some of my best teachers. They endured years of rejection, moving forward each year with hope and confidence in the ultimate end game. They really get why they chose medicine and they identify very clearly with the profession, warts and all. They are also passionate about sharing their love of medicine and creating remarkable pedagogical experiences without exception.

Failure should be our teacher, not our undertaker.
Failure is delay, not defeat. It is a temporary detour, not
a dead end. Failure is something we can avoid only by
saying nothing, doing nothing, and being nothing.
- DENIS WAITLEY

I want you to know that rejection is perfectly acceptable. I was personally rejected from medical school twice between 2006 and 2012. In many cases, it is temporary. My most convicted motivation to do what I needed to do to get into medical school did not take shape until I figured out why I wanted to be a doctor. My graduate degree, a Master's of Public Health with a concentration in Global Health, was transformational, both personally and professionally. I found out that the study of addiction could hold my attention more than any other area of work. I interned at the United Nations. I wrote a final thesis of which I am very proud. I was able to develop a personal ethos for working with very vulnerable people and my own worldview about the nature of our social problems was rendered so much more nuanced by my work and studies. My thesis research looked at the role of social capital in shaping the relationships between physicians and women who sell sex and do high risk drugs in Vancouver's downtown east side. I spent a lot of time sitting in clinic waiting rooms, talking to patients and providers, thinking about the health system, the built environment, and the social policy ecosystem in which so many people are made more sick. Medicine became more real for me during that experience than any other time in my life. But I also saw so many other leverage points, places in the system that I could work to make change.

Over four years, I finished graduate school and was recruited to an elite government policy leader program with the Public Health Agency of Canada's Health Determinants and Global Initiatives Division. I had become really passionate about public health systems and I was so excited to land this permanent, well-paying, exciting job in Ottawa at the age of 24. Except it was literally the worst. I was so under-worked, under-stimulated and caged-in by a political environment that precluded real action on the social determinants of health. My colleagues were wonderful, but I was bored out of my mind. For the first time in my life, I asked myself, "What is it that you want to DO every day?" I had thought a lot about what I wanted to BE but nothing really specific ever came up so I always just followed topics that I thought were of real importance, like social justice and public health. I realized I wanted to be in relationships with people. I wanted to help solve problems on a daily basis. I wanted to help people with their bodies and examine how they could be well. I wanted to work at a community level to help people through their stories of love, grief, sickness and triumph. I wanted to be a local leader. That is when I figured out that I wanted to be a doctor. Finally, I had answered the most important question. This was the best motivation I could have possibly hoped for in order to make medical school happen for me.

I signed up to write my MCAT in July 2010. I decided three weeks before the exam date to actually write the test because I wanted to apply in the coming fall. I couldn't take time off from work, so I just decided to write the verbal section and apply again to McMaster and NOSM. I completely guessed through the biological and physical sciences section and nailed the verbal and writing sections. I submitted my second application from Ottawa to NOSM and McMaster. These were the only schools to which I was eligible to apply given my lack of prerequisite courses, my terrible MCAT scores and the fact that I am not fluent in French.

It was a challenge to submit a medical school application three years out from undergraduate studies. First of all, I had almost 10 years' worth of extra-curricular activities to pare down to 48 entries for the OMSAS autobiographical sketch. My undergraduate professors advised me that I should try to get letters of reference from graduate school because it had been so long since I was an undergraduate student. I struggled to figure out if I should be emphasizing my undergraduate life or my graduate life. The correct answer is probably both. Tracking down verifiers was a big job. It took a lot more time to put together my second application and I recommend anyone in the same boat try to be prepared.

While I was waiting for decisions, I changed up my career and moved to Afghanistan to do some grassroots work with an NGO. I went for less than half of the salary and I don't regret a thing. I found out in Afghanistan that McMaster didn't want to interview me but NOSM did. I flew home to interview in Thunder Bay, and was in the bazaar at a carpet seller stall when I got the email saying I had been rejected again by NOSM. I submitted my third application to McMaster and NOSM in the fall of 2011 from Afghanistan. It was an identical application to the last. My statistics were identical. My approach to CASPer was exactly the same as the year before.

There were two sets of challenges to my third application cycle. The first set was related to Afghanistan. The Internet was decent, but not always excellent. The country was in increasing turmoil in advance of the US pullout. There were more and more attacks on Kabul, most of which reached a fever pitch in 2014 and 2015. I was working 14 or more hours in a day with a lot of travelling, meetings and a lot of being very tired.

The second set was related to my mindset. I had no reason to believe I was going to get into medical school. NOSM had rejected me twice after meeting me and McMaster hadn't even wanted to meet me. Why would this year be any different? I assumed I would not be accepted to join the Class of 2015 and was already planning my next application. My good friend – who was studying at the University of Toronto's medical school - said to me, "you need to show up to the game," meaning that I need to show that I am willing to tick the boxes of a medical school candidate. I needed to show consistency and commitment.

So, fine, I thought. I left my budding career in international development - and a country I was coming to really love - to take organic chemistry at the University of Ottawa, get more prerequisites to apply to more schools in Canada and rewrite the MCAT. My backup plan - I needed one, at age 28 - was to get accepted to medical school in the Caribbean but defer for one year to take a job with the Ministry of Counter Narcotics in Afghanistan, which would have paid for the entire thing. I know this sounds crazy but here's the thing: I knew why I wanted to be a doctor and nothing was going to hold me back.

In the organic chemistry lectures (I had an excellent story-telling professor), I sat with 17 year olds in their first or second year of university. I couldn't see the slides very well because I was getting old. I sat in the front row of that lecture hall for four months, turning molecules into stories, and finished with an A+ in first year organic chemistry at the University of Ottawa. I found out in January that I got an interview at McMaster but none at NOSM, and within six weeks of finishing organic chemistry, I found out I was accepted to McMaster University's Michael

G. DeGroote School of Medicine in the Class of 2015. If I hadn't been accepted, I would have applied the year after, to more schools. And the year after. And the year after.

Preparing for Interviews

For the first two interviews at NOSM, I basically winged them. I read up on MMI best practices and did some practice questions with friends. Then I just hoped for the best. When I got the interview at McMaster in January 2012, I knew that it was like a little gift from the universe. I had to be prepared. I hired a company that specializes in interview preparation to break down my performance in mock interviews and show me how to put it back together smoothly, clearly and effectively. I practiced for days. I was relentless in my preparation for that interview because I knew I had all of the raw materials to do very well. I have a stellar vocabulary, I am an extrovert who speaks to all sorts of people all the time, I have a vast well of life and professional experiences to speak on, I have a graduate degree in the content from which many MMI questions are drawn. I argue well and cooperate in teams. The coaching represented clarity and finesse and I do not regret paying for that service.

What are the keys to success?

I believe that there are four keys to success for getting into medical school. They apply equally to traditional and non-traditional applicants:

Prepare and plan. Chart out your courses to fourth year during first year. Be open to change as your interests evolve. If you're late to preparing and planning, start now. I started after graduate school, which was almost too late but not quite.

Take risks with life, not with your application. Be strategically daring. Don't do work that makes you physically ill. On your application, tick all the boxes. Don't give them a reason to toss your application. Grades first!

Believe that you're going to be a doctor but also believe that it is going to take a lot of work. Be teachable with each application cycle. And be even more teachable in medical school.

Don't fall apart when you're rejected. Just keep going. Rejection isn't a statement on your quality of character so don't take it personally.

Case Six: Daniel E. Wang, B.Eng., MS, MBA, MD(c)
Bachelor of Engineering (McGill)
Master of Science (University of Michigan)
Master of Business Administration (University of Michigan)
GPA: 3.90
MCAT: Physical 11 (128), CARS 11 (128) Biological 11 (128)

My journey to medical school was probably atypical compared to most. Not only was I considered a mature student (becoming a physician was a second career choice), but I was also giving up a successful management consulting practice (to the surprise of many) to do so, as well as starting a family at the same time.

My decision to pursue medical studies came later in life; it wasn't until I lost my dad to cancer that I really started rethinking my career and the kind of impact I wanted to leave on society.

After much personal deliberation, conversations with family, friends and physicians, as well as research into medical programs and career opportunities, I decided to give it a shot. It was by no means an easy decision but the process effectively involved five key steps, as described below.

Step 1: Research schools and eligibility
My primary consideration in school selection was location. Due to family commitments (a full-time working spouse and young daughter on the way), I knew I had to be as close to our home in Toronto as possible: as far I considered it at the time, first tier schools were U of T and McMaster, second tier schools were any within a 5-hour drive, i.e.,

Western, Queen's, Ottawa and McGill. With this short list of schools, I then looked at personal eligibility requirements. I ruled out McGill because I didn't meet their timeline for completing basic science requirements (despite having completed these courses at McGill during undergrad) and I didn't want to retake three sets of full-year courses. I ruled out Ottawa based on my belief, rightly or wrongly, that they were not particularly receptive to mature Anglophone students (especially with my two master's degrees and decade long professional career). I ruled out Western due to their high MCAT biology cut-off (I had a minimal biology background).

Step 2: Select schools and take prerequisites
Looking at the requirements for the three remaining schools (Queen's, McMaster and Toronto), I realized I not only had to write the MCAT but also had to take both organic chemistry and biochemistry (I had taken general sciences in my first year at McGill before switching into engineering, during which I also took several humanities courses). I took biochemistry and organic chemistry in the evening while working during the day and studied for the MCAT through an online prep course during the summer before applications were due.

Step 3: Finalize and confirm references
Knowing I needed three references (at least one academic) plus a specific master's program reference for U of T, I quickly identified six potential references (four from my professional career and two from my masters' program). I analyzed each potential reference's ability to speak to my personal and professional skill sets and capabilities and mapped each to their ability to speak to any or all of the seven attributes of the CanMEDS framework. I then narrowed this list to the final four references based on coverage of the CanMEDS attributes as well as my perception of their individual writing skills. I asked all four references and all but one said yes right away. The fourth questioned me substantially on why I wanted to become a physician at this stage of my career before agreeing to the request. I honestly believe

that my ability to articulate and convince her of my desire to practice medicine probably made her an even stronger reference than the other three.

Step 4: Start written application process (bio, essays, letter requests and transcript requests)

While taking night class, I also started working on my written applications, notably preparing my autobiographic sketch, requesting transcripts from universities, and reviewing essay requirements. I also created a master project plan of to-dos and timelines for each school so that I could keep track of what activities were due at what time. This schedule also allowed me to plan for sufficient time for application reviews. To prepare my sketch, I created a spreadsheet of all possible activities, dates, locations, achievements and possible verifiers going all the way back to my last year of high school. Because of my numerous professional and post-graduate experiences, I knew I would have to eliminate many of them to meet the limits of the application requirements. It was at this point that I hired BeMo to help me with my sketch as well as review drafts of essays. My essay writing process involved reviewing a few books on medical school applications as well as writing many drafts that were not only reviewed by BeMo, but also trusted family members and physician friends. After receiving feedback on my sketch and essays, I spent substantial time formatting both to meet the online technical requirements of OMSAS, (e.g., checking character counts and limits, formatting and spacing, as well as of course grammar and spelling). I did all of this offline where it was easier to keep track of edits and changes so that I could just copy and paste into the online system at the end.

Step 5: Prepare for CASPer and interviews

I actually found this last step personally easiest of the five steps. With my work and academic background, I had interviewed for numerous jobs, internships and scholastic programs and had also conducted interviews myself in such settings. Thus, I focused this time studying medical news and events, healthcare systems and politics, recent medical court cases, and of course, medical ethics. I include preparing for CASPer as part of this step, as I believed CASPer would cover similar material as the in-person interviews. For both CASPer and interviews, I prepared a series of study notes summarizing the topics above and subscribed to several medical news feeds and blogs to read while riding transit to and from work. And of course, performed lots of mock interviews and CASPer practice tests with BeMo.

Final Thoughts

Based on good but less-than-stellar MCAT and GPA scores, I like to believe it was professional maturity, strong reference letters, and impressive interviews that enabled me to receive offers of acceptance into all three schools. But I also firmly believe there is quite a bit of luck in the admissions process (have you ever read a CV on two different days and had two different opinions of it?). I consider myself incredibly fortunate not only to have made it through the process but to have had the amazing support of my spouse, family and friends along the way. However, if there is one piece of advice that I can share with prospective applicants: start your application early and don't think you can do it all on your own: no matter how bright, articulate, and organized you are, you may be surprised what a second set of eyes may find!

Case Seven: Dr. Janet McMordie B.Sc., M.Sc., M.D. (Family Medicine – Sports Medicine)

Bachelor of Science in Human Kinetics (St Francis Xavier)
Master of Science in Kinesiology (Western)
GPA: 3.95
MCAT: Physical 14 (131), CARS 10 (127), Biological 9 (125)

I started thinking about medical school when I was in high school. I took a fitness class in Gr 12 instead of the normal sports-based physical education class and it sparked my interest in Kinesiology and the science of exercise. I did my undergrad at St Francis Xavier University, a small school in Nova Scotia. I loved being in a small program because there was a lot of one-on-one time with professors and a tight-knit collegial atmosphere. No competition! I loved my courses and my GPA showed it. I was so fascinated by everything I was learning. If there is one piece of advice I can give, it is to study what you enjoy, not what you think will get you into medical school. Your enjoyment will be reflected in your GPA as well as your personality!

Memorable undergrad extracurricular activities: campus police officer; campus tour guide; student council member; Just 4 Kicks (after school recreation program for kids with disabilities)

I wrote the MCAT in the summer between my 3rd and 4th year and did terrible! It was very frustrating and I turned my focus from medical school to research. I did an honors research project that was very successful. I presented at some top conferences in the states and had my research featured on msnbc.com, Women's Health magazine, and several well-known fitness blogs.

I went to Western University for my Master's in Kinesiology. I enjoyed doing my Master's but realized soon into the process that I didn't enjoy the research aspect of it as much as I enjoyed the interaction with my research participants! I remember one of my supervisors noticing this and said to me: "you know Janet, you might consider medical school" (UGH FINE!) So my focus went back to medical school!!

I worked as a fitness instructor for an incredible group of retired researchers at the university (who gave me my stethoscope when I got in!) and volunteered in the orthopedic department of the hospital. I re-wrote the MCAT and did significantly better than the last time but my 9 in the biology section prevented me from applying to a couple of schools. I applied to McMaster and McMaster only with the plan to re-write the MCAT again if I wasn't successful. The application process was fairly easy for me with just one school! McMaster has several essay-like questions as part of their application. My Mom was a huge help editing my answers and I believe one of the main reasons I got an interview! I made my essay responses as personal and as unique as possible, highlighting some of my more "interesting" extracurricular activities (camp counsellor at a summer camp for children/teens who are HIV positive, organizing a battle of the bands), ones that I thought would make me stand out among the masses of applicants. It must've worked because I was offered an interview!

Knowing I only had one shot and a very slim shot as an out of province applicant (I'm from BC and McMaster only accepts about 10 people from out of province), I did a lot of interview prep through the university career center. I found it so helpful. I did two practice MMIs and even had an interview session videotaped so I could watch myself! I practiced with my friends and by myself in front of the mirror. I had my CV memorized with lots of personal anecdotes at the ready!

I love interviews and I LOVED my MMI experience. I found it so fun. I don't remember being nervous, just excited. I felt really confident with nearly all of my stations. There weren't any surprises and I know I felt that way because of the preparation I did. At almost all of the stations, I was able to talk about personal experiences that related to the question asked. I remember leaving the interview knowing I had a good chance of getting a spot.

I know my experience with this process is quite unique. One and done! I feel very privileged to have had the experience I had. If there is any piece of advice I can give, its DO WHAT YOU LOVE. Never do anything you aren't passionate about because you think it will help you get into medical school because your lack of passion shows...truly.

When I'm interviewing applicants these days, I look for that passion. Its very easy to spot and difficult to fake.

I am currently doing a fellowship in sport and exercise medicine at McMaster which was my dream since starting medical school and learning that sports medicine was an option! Throughout medical school and residency, I did several electives in sports medicine across the country and attended every conference I could find! I also volunteered to do medical coverage at numerous sporting events. Sports medicine has become quite competitive. In my year, there were eight applicants for one spot at McMaster. I applied to five fellowship programs and was offered a spot at 4, waitlisted at one. McMaster was my top choice and I happily accepted!

Prior to my fellowship, I did my residency in family medicine at McMaster as well. I applied to three schools but ranked McMaster first.

I also got my first choice of location which was wonderful! I had done a broad range of electives in my clerkship that were applicable to family medicine (adolescent medicine and psychiatry to name a few). The interview process again, like medical school, was really fun! It was more relaxed than medical school. I felt like I was having a nice chat with every interviewer! I filled my answers with lots of personal anecdotes from my medical school experience and left each school feeling very confident!

Medical school is not for the faint of heart or the indecisive. I know now that I wasn't ready for medical school after my undergrad and, looking back on it I'm happy my first MCAT score prevented me from applying (my parents knew I wasn't ready then yet either...parents are always right!). I don't think I was mature enough. I think I wanted medical school because everyone else did and it was something I had told everyone I wanted to do. I wasn't doing it for myself. Doing my masters was the turning point for me. I matured a ton in those two years. I worked hard, travelled a lot, and (super corny) did a ton of soul searching. Once you're in medical school, your life as you knew it before, is over. You are in a whole different world, you learn a whole different language, and your entire social circle will change. You won't relate to people you knew prior to medical school the same anymore. You see things and experience things that nobody understands except for those who have gone/ are going through it themselves. It can be very frustrating and depressing so you need to choose medical school for YOURSELF. Think really hard about your choice. Medical school and being a doctor is the most rewarding thing I have ever done. I love being a doctor. It has been such a long, exhausting, expensive journey to get to where I am, but I know I wouldn't want to be doing anything else. Make sure you feel the same way.

CHAPTER X

BeMo's TOP 8 RULES for Getting into Med School

As you've probably gathered by now, getting into Med School is no walk in the park. It's a juggling act that consists of sacrificed weekends, long hours of volunteering, mental and physical exhaustion, all topped off with the application preparation. And if you've followed and read the previous chapters properly, you should have a good understanding that preparation is key. Medical school acceptance is hard, and looking at the official statistics reveals that the success rate in U.S and Canada could be as low as 2%. Every year eager applicants with high MCAT and GPA scores get the dreaded rejection letter, while diversified applicants get the sought out acceptance letter. WHY? You must plan smart and in advance!

Let's look at three common myths about the medical school application process:

MYTH 1: "You must enroll in a pre-med program"

Applicants often think that you must enroll in a medical related program; life sciences, health sciences or a premed program. There is nothing further from the truth. The majority of medical schools DO NOT care what program you take in undergrad. In fact, their main objective is to ensure that you have taken the prerequisite courses, and performed well academically, regardless of the program of study. An applicant with a diverse educational background is actually preferred.

MYTH 2: "You must attend a 'brand name' university"

Most applicants feel that if they attend a prestigious school, such as Harvard or the University of Toronto, they will have higher chances of acceptance. However, much like your program of study, medical school only cares if you performed well academically and meet the requirements. Moreover, sometimes attending a notable school may hurt you as an applicant, since there is greater competition, bigger classrooms leading to less interaction with the professors, etc. all lending to poor relationships and weak reference letters.

MYTH 3: "All that matters is your grades & MCAT"

It is important to reiterate that having a high GPA and MCAT score does not guarantee an acceptance into medical school. As statistics indicate, a significant amount of applicants with such scores are rejected annually. Why, well because medical schools are looking for candidates who have demonstrated other important factors such as; strong emotional intelligence and non-cognitive abilities. This is why applicants have to adhere to lengthy detailed applications, essays, personal letters, and even interviews.

Now, let's looks at BeMo's Top 8 Rules for getting into Med school:

RULE #1: Students that plan in advance are 10 times more likely to get in

According to a BeMo independent study, students that plan ahead are 10 times more likely to get in *the first time* they apply. As previously examined, the application process is lengthy and as such requires proper planning. Therefore, it is crucial that you plan well in advance.

RULE #2: You must have a plan of action to stand out from early undergrad/late high school years

Applicants must be involved in appropriate activities both academically and non academically. Diversifying your application allows you to stand out, while at the same time suggesting to the admission panel that you are a well-rounded candidate.

RULE #3: Be wary of online forums and pre-med clubs

Be aware, online forums are usually filled with inaccurate information from unknown sources and some online forums actively seek 'sponsors' to generate revenue giving certain organizations a dedicated medium to expand their agenda rather than actively share genuine information to help their members. Additionally, most pre-med clubs have exclusive financial partnerships with various companies in exchange for access to student's information and emails, which serves as a marketing strategy. As a result, members are restricted to the perspectives shared by these clubs, thus limiting students' ability to make an informed decision. Moreover, it is important to note, if you plan on standing out, then it would not make sense to do what everyone else is doing, this would only make you a generic applicant. Therefore, if you use the 'tips' you found an online forum or a premed club you can be sure that another 700 students are also using the same exact 'tips', which guarantees that you will not stand out. This is the reason BeMo often turns down offers to sponsor premed forums and clubs.

RULE #4: You must follow your PASSION!

It is critical that you explore your commitment level before diving head-first. When you are whole-heartedly committed to something, then you are more apt to try harder, and perform better. Thus, you will do well academically and achieve the GPA you are looking for.

RULE #5: You can enroll in ANY program/university

As previously discussed, it is not essential to enroll in a medical program or a prestigious school. As long as you perform extremely well academically and meet all the requirements set out by faculties of medicine, you are qualified, if not preferred.

RULE #6: You must select appropriate non-academic activities & referees

You must recall that gaining admissions is about demonstrating your abilities. Medical programs want to know that you are a well-rounded person, who possesses non-cognitive skills and emotional intelligence. In order to advance these abilities and advance your application, you need to get involved in activities outside of academics. These activities will serve to further your application chances and will be used as evidence to showcase whether you possess such strong abilities.

RULE #7: You MUST get rid of ALL your "Plan Bs"

Yes, this might sound untraditional, but having plan B's like graduate school or other professional programs weakens your chances of admissions. Having such back up plans means you are not whole-heartedly committed to the process and negatively impacts your mindset. If that is the case, it is pivotal that you reexamine where you want to spend the next four years of your life. Importantly, if you do commit and do all the things we have discussed in this book, you will have plenty of other options to explore if medical school doesn't work out at the end.

RULE #8: You must invest MORE time & resources prior to applications + no magic pill

Why? If you recall, we have on numerous occasions suggested that planning in advance is essential, and doing all the right things before you apply is important so you can demonstrate that you have done your due diligence to posses strong non cognitive abilities and emotional intelligence. You will need to prove that you have taken sufficient amount of time investigating the profession; increasing your knowledge through various non-academic activities, all while developing your abilities as an applicant, and as an individual.

In addition, it is also important to note that there is no magic pill to bypass or win the process. The application process in all of its entirety requires rigorous work and strategic planning.

And here is how BeMo can help!

Now that you have been fully equipped with BeMo's "myths and facts", it is critical that you begin your planning to a successful application, and most importantly your admissions to medical school! We would wish you luck, but as we know by now, luck is not a main part of the equation; you are!

CHAPTER XI

Resources and Useful tools

(http://bemoacademicconsulting.com/premed-resources)

This final chapter is designed to serve as a resource guide to help you plan and apply to medical school once the time has come. These resources were comprised with the aid of BeMo's team of admissions experts and we believe that you will find them useful.

Note that the resources provided are divided into distinct sections. These sections include, information on medical schools and their statistics in the US and Canada, strategies for medical school planning, application components (i.e. personal statements, ABS, CASPer, etc.), interviews, and more.

To gain access to these resources visit:

http://bemoacademicconsulting.com/premed-resources

Section one: Resources for the planning stages & writing the MCAT

BeMo's medical school planning program

How to select extracurricular & volunteer activities to increase your chances of acceptance to med school – BeMo blog

How to select the best verifiers and referees and ask for reference letters – BeMo blog

Will volunteering abroad really increase your chances of admissions to med school – BeMo blog

Four fatal errors that got me rejected from medical school – Twice – And how to avoid them – BeMo blog

How to get into med school as a non-traditional and/or mature applicant – BeMo blog

How to get into ANY medical school – BeMo blog

How to maximize your university grades without turning into a bookworm – BeMo blog

BeMo OMSAS GPA Conversion calculator what to do if your GPA is low – BeMo blog

Everything you need to know about American medical school applications and processes - AAMC website
Everything you need to know about Medical School Admission Requirements – USA

Required Pre-medical coursework and competencies organized by school – USA

Timeline for Application/Admission to Medical School – USA

Pre-Med coursework worksheet - USA – *allows for organization and tracking of pre-requisite courses* -

Factors to weigh before applying worksheet – *Use form to identify and assess schools to which you want to apply* – USA

Information on all medical schools within Canada

Ontario Medical School Application Services – Canada – *Everything you need to know about the application process in Ontario, Canada*

CanMed Framework provides an in-depth analysis of the qualities and characteristics sought after and required by medical schools in

AMCAS GPA conversion instructions and charts

Official AAMC MCAT website – Everything you need to know about the MCAT

e-MCAT practice: The official MCAT practice site -

Section two: application and applying
BeMo Application Review Program

Sample Personal Statements/Essays - USA

Sample Short Essays – Canada

Sample Autobiographical Sketches – Canada

Sample AMCAS work/activity section - USA

AMCAS Application Tips – What to include & exclude in your application – BeMo blog

An inside guide to the Ontario Medical School Application Services (OMSAS) – BeMo blog

The top 10 mistakes you must avoid in your med school essays and personal statements – BeMo blog

The top 11 essential qualities to include in your med school essays – BeMo blog

How to choose the "right" med school? – BeMo blog

U of T med school brief personal essay tips – BeMo blog

How to make your OMSAS sketch stand out? – BeMo blog

How to make your AMCAS ABS entries stand out? – BeMo blog

How to write the perfect AMCAS personal statement? – BeMo blog

Top 5 reasons 90% of medical school applicants get rejected and how to avoid them – BeMo blog

Top 4 ingredients of a successful medical school application – BeMo blog

Best time to start your medical school application – BeMo blog

Section three: CASPer
BeMo's CASPer SIM™ tests (CASPer simulation) and CASPer prep program

BeMo's ultimate guide for the CASPer test – CASPer test prep tips, strategies & sample questions -

Top five tips for acing your CASPer Test – BeMo blog

Former CASPer Test evaluator reveals her top CASPer prep tips! – BeMo blog

CASPer & MMI prep myths busted! The "secrets" admissions committees would never want you to know – BeMo blog

Sample CASPer scenario + questions & expert response – BeMo blog

Shocking McMaster med school statistics and proven strategies to prepare for CASPer – BeMo blog

Section four: Interview
BeMo med school interview preparation program

BeMo MMI prep program

BeMo resource guide for medical school interviews

How to answer the dreaded med school interview question: "Tell me about yourself?" – BeMo blog

How to prepare on your interview day – Here's our top 8 tips – BeMo blog

How do I answer the interview question: What is your greatest limitation? Or What's your greatest weakness? – BeMo blog

How to ace medical school interview policy type questions – BeMo blog

How to ace your panel, traditional or conversational med school interview – BeMo blog

How to ace the multiple mini interview (MMI) acting station - BeMo blog

How to ace the multiple mini interview (MMI) collaboration/teamwork stations – BeMo blog

Sample MMI questions - BeMo blogs

Former med school admissions interviewer reveals her best strategies to ace the most common types of medical school interview questions – BeMo blog

Sample difficult med school interview question and expert response – BeMo blog

Former MMI evaluator reveals her top MMI prep tips! – BeMo blog

How to prepare for your MMI? – BeMo blog

Sample MMI question + expert analysis and response – BeMo blog

Ultimate guide to the Modified Personal Interview (MPI) – BeMo blog

Ultimate guide to medical school interview questions – BeMo blog

Medical school interviews and the birth of the MMI – BeMo blog`

Made in the USA
Lexington, KY
05 June 2018